# Bodybuilding: From Heavy Duty to SuperSlow

## Evolutionary Strategies for Building Maximum Muscle

**Craig Cecil**

# Bodybuilding: From Heavy Duty to SuperSlow – Evolutionary Strategies for Building Maximum Muscle

ISBN: 978-0-9847414-5-8
ISBN: 978-0-9847414-4-1 (ebook)

Manufactured in the United States of America

Trademarked names may appear in this book. Rather than use a trademark symbol with every occurrence of a trademarked name, we use the names only in an editorial fashion and to the benefit of the trademark owner, with no intention of infringement of the trademark.

**Warning:** Before beginning any exercise program, consult with your physician to ensure that you are in proper health. This book does not provide medical or therapeutic advice; you should obtain medical advice from your healthcare practitioner. Before starting any new program, check with your doctor, especially if you have a specific physical problem or are taking medication. No liability is assumed by the author or publisher for any of the information contained herein.

Cover design by Jaclyn Urlahs.
Cover photo by Nikolay Suslov (NiDerLander).

# Contents

# Thanks!

This book is dedicated to all those going on the journey, whether beginner or seasoned veteran. It's you versus you and the ride of a lifetime.

Thanks also to those whose words and experiences educated and inspired me over the decades, including: Arnold, Joe, Franco, Frank, Lou, Larry, Dave, Mike, Lee, Chris, Stuart, Skip, Clarence, Dan and countless others. Some of you I've met and talked to personally—others, I hear your words still to this day.

Finally, thanks to Leslie and Mitch for helping with the editing of this book. This is a better book because of you.

# Tell Me What You Think

I'm always interested in getting feedback on my books. Please send your comments and suggestions to:

books@runningdeersoftware.com

# Preface

Millions of individuals across the world engage in weight training activities every day, many in the hope of building bigger, stronger and more muscular bodies. Many reach their goal—many do not. If you look at a cross-section of these individuals, they use various approaches to weight training. Which work? Which work best? Why do some train this way and others that?

This book presents over a dozen weight training systems developed over the past century. While most of these systems are geared towards bodybuilding, some have wider applicability to powerlifting and Olympic lifting. I make no overall judgments regarding each system—I leave it up to you to learn about each, try them for at least 6-8 weeks and then make your own decision as to their effectiveness, based on your body's response and your goals. I will however, point out where various systems align or diverge, things to watch out for, and how they stack up against each other.

I hope after reading this book, you will have gained wider knowledge, application and appreciation for the vast possibilities in weight training and building muscle. Along the way, I'll throw in a history lesson or two—the barbells and dumbbells you hold in your hands and the way you use them have stories to tell.

Remember, the journey and the relationships you build with yourself and others is the reward. Onward.

*Craig*

Westminster, MD
July 2012

# Introduction

Progressive resistance training and the systems developed for this activity date back over two thousand years, from the days of Milo, the five-time Olympic Games winner in ancient Greece, to the efforts of millions of individuals throughout gyms, schools and homes around the world.

Over time, numerous weight training systems have emerged and evolved—some birthing others, a few rejecting the past and boldly striking out on their own. However, all of these systems share a common goal: to maximize and overcome our bodies amazing ability to adapt and survive whatever we challenge it with.

Which concepts, methodology or systems should you use?

This book takes you through a historical tour, explaining the evolution and details of the most popular weight training systems developed over the past century, so you can make your own decision regarding which work best for you. Along the way, you'll gain the basic knowledge and understanding of each in order to try them yourself. It's extremely important to find the optimal workout methodology for your body, since the higher the quality of muscular work you can generate, the greater the effect on your body and the faster you will progress toward your goals. So, don't be a lemming simply following the hordes in the gym—discover your options and chart your own course.

Here are the weight training systems on the journey we'll take. You'll get the most benefit from reading through them in order, since most build upon past discoveries—however; feel free to skip to ones that particularly interest you.

## The 1930s

General Principles of Exercise

## The 1950s

Volume Training

## The 1960s

PHA Training
High Intensity Training (HIT)
Periodization

## The 1970s

The Bulgarian Method
Pre-Exhaustion
Heavy Duty

## The 1980s

The Weider System
The Hardgainer Method
SuperSlow
Holistic Training
Power Factor Training

## The 1990s

Positions of Flexion (POF)
Static Contraction Training

Each of these weight training systems can be classified by two factors—
**volume and intensity**.

*Volume* relates to how many sets and exercises you perform during a workout, as well as how often you work out during a week, month, or year. *Intensity* is defined as the amount of energy you expend or muscular activation you affect within a given period of time. If you can do more work in a shorter period of time, exhausting more muscle fibers, then your workout intensity will be higher than what you were previously doing. Of course, intensity is relative. What's intense to one person may be a walk in the park to another.

Let's take a look at where each system falls into place with volume and intensity.

## High-Volume, Low Intensity

Volume Training
PHA Training
Holistic Training

## High-Volume, High Intensity

The Bulgarian Method
Pre-Exhaustion
Power Factor Training
Points of Flexion (POF)

## Low-Volume, High-Intensity

Heavy Duty
High-Intensity Training (HIT)
The Hardgainer Method
SuperSlow
Static Contraction Training

## All of the Above

Periodization
The Weider System

Most individuals spend most of their time in the high-volume, low intensity world. The biggest changes come when you break into one of the other quadrants.

## Overload and Intensity

Each of these weight training systems manipulates volume and intensity by adjusting one or more of the following variables:

- Exercise selection

- Performance technique

- Number of repetitions

- Amount of weight

- Repetition tempo

- Range of motion

- Rest intervals between sets

- Number of sets performed per muscle group

- Total number of sets performed during the workout

- Training frequency—number of training sessions per day and per week

- The amount of eccentric (lowering of the weight) work the muscles are required to perform

By increasing exercise intensity, you affect muscle overload. There are several general methods for overloading a muscle, each with distinct results:

| Method of Overload | Primary Result |
| --- | --- |
| Increase weight | Strength |
| Increase repetitions | Muscular Endurance |
| Increase movement speed | Explosiveness |
| Increase duration of effort per rep (time under load) | Vascularity and Muscular Endurance |
| Increase number of maximum efforts (1RM) | Strength endurance and strength |
| Increase frequency of sets/decrease rest time between sets | Cardiovascular and muscular endurance |
| Increase number of exercises per workout | Cardiovascular and muscular endurance |
| Increase number of workouts per week | Cardiovascular and muscular endurance |

Additionally, each of the weight training systems I'll discuss manipulates the methods for increasing intensity and overload by taking sides on the following issues:

- Free weights vs. Machines
- Compound vs. Isolation Movements
- Few vs. Many Exercises
- High vs. Low Reps
- Single vs. Multiple Sets
- Long vs. Short Training Sessions
- Short vs. Long Rests between Sets
- Slow vs. Fast Tempos (Contraction Speed)
- Full vs. Partial Range of Motion

In the remainder of this book, you'll learn how all of these factors are used to construct the basic tenets of each weight training system. But first, let's look at the general principles of resistance training which are common to all of these systems.

# General Principles

Before the turn of the 20th century, no formalized methods or principles of resistance training were recorded and generally accepted. Circus strongmen and travelling strength performers such as Donald Dinnie, John Grun, and Louis Cyr, closely guarded the "secrets" to their size and strength in order to protect their livelihood and enhance the spectacle. Lifting wagon wheels overhead was clearly not the norm, attracted large audiences and paid very well.

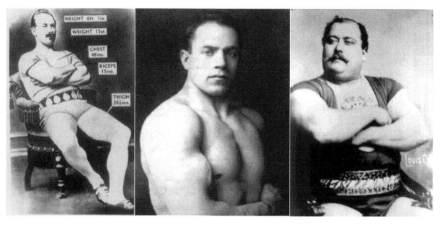

*From left to right: Donald Dinnie, John Grun, and Louis Cyr*

It wasn't until the Hungarian endocrinologist, Dr. Hans Selye, finally published *The Stress of Life* in 1956 that the principles of progressive resistance were first formalized and accepted. Dr. Selye noted in his work that exercise was a primary form of stress—thus the floodgates were open. Selye began publishing his results in 1936, while at Canada's McGill University—one Canadian in particular paid attention to this academic work and began laying the foundation for a layman's interpretation that he could build upon, promote and sell to the world—Joe Weider.

Seyle identified several of the modern principles of progressive resistance training which are common throughout the various training systems presented in this book. Some of the systems recognize and model all of these principles, while others emphasize one or two of the principles specifically. Let's look at each of the general principles.

## The Principle of Individual Differences

Each trainer has different abilities, structures, lever attributes, and muscle fiber composition, and therefore responds somewhat differently to any given system of training. Consequently, consider these individual differences when selecting or performing within any given training system.

You've seen this in practice. Tall people generally have a harder time squatting or deadlifting. Individuals with barrel-shaped chests seem to be able to bench press effectively at will. Others with shallow ribcages and wide clavicles feel most pressing movements in their shoulders, not their chest. Here, the kind and cruel duality of genetics largely dictates the potential size of your chest or the width of your shoulders.

## The Overcompensation Principle

The body will overcompensate from stress on the muscles by growing bigger and stronger muscles. It really does boil down to this simplicity.

## The Overload Principle

To make your body overcompensate, you must stress (overload) your muscles beyond what they have done before. Milo, the 6th century Olympic wrestler, is the embodiment of this principle. As lore tells us, part of his training consisted of lifting and carrying a newborn bull, repeating the feat daily as the bull grew to maturity. Now, that's progressive overload.

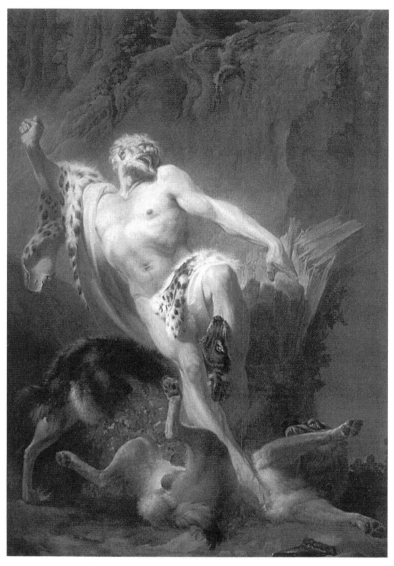

*Milo of Croton by Joseph-Benoit Suvee*

What's not progressive overload is seeing the same person come into the gym and perform the same exercises, at the same pace, in the same order, with the same weight, and the same grip time after time. Their body doesn't change, because none of the underlying training variables changed in order to increase intensity and overload. Now, that's a waste of time. Change *something!*

## The SAID Principle

SAID is the acronym for Specific Adaptation to Imposed Demands. Stressing a muscle beyond normal limits will cause adaptation (growth response) to occur.

Here's a simple example. Let's say that the heaviest barbell that you routinely pick up and hold in your workout is 100 lbs. Now, if you start holding a 150 lb. barbell (just pick it off a rack slightly and hold it for a minute) every day for a couple months, what will happen? Your body will say, "Hey, I guess I've got to hold this really heavy barbell every day, so I might as well make my forearm muscles bigger so I can handle it easily because I don't like to work this hard". This is also the reason why your calves get bigger (yes, even a little) if you put on more body weight. You're propelling a bigger you forward with each step. (I hate to say it—but some of the biggest calves you'll ever see are on obese people. As their fat accumulated, their calves compensated.)

## The Use/Disuse Principle

The muscles will hypertrophy (grow) with use and atrophy (shrink) if you don't use them or use them infrequently. You've probably heard this referred to as "use it or lose it."

## The GAS Principle

GAS is the acronym for General Adaptation Syndrome. Selye formalized that since exercise is a form of stress, the body reacts to stress in three stages:

1. **Alarm Stage**
   The body recognizes and begins to make changes to account for the stress factor (e.g., muscle overload). A temporary drop in performance due to stiffness and muscle soreness often characterizes this stage. In *The Stress of Life*, Selye notes, "the alarm response of the body is directly proportionate to the intensity of the aggression." This core concept is the central tenet of the Heavy Duty system, as well as other permutations of high-intensity training I'll discuss in subsequent sections.

2. **Resistance Stage**
   The body adapts to the stress by making changes. For example, when you apply stress to a muscle through resistance training, the body adapts by increasing the size of the muscle to deal with increased weight loads.

3. **Exhaustion Stage**

You reach this when the body is overwhelmed by stress and can't adapt in time. This causes over-training. As you'll see, many of the systems in this book attempt to avoid this stage by manipulating the frequency of training. The key is to apply stress via exercise without overwhelming your body's recovery ability and causing over-training. That's why you shouldn't work the same muscles every day. Therefore, for constant adaptation to occur, follow periods of high-intensity training with periods of low intensity training (see *Cycle Training Principle* and *Periodization*). In reality, it's often a razor's edge you'll walk between coaxing adaptation while avoiding exhaustion (or injury). Master this, and you'll unlock the key to continual progress.

# The Specificity Principle

The body gets stronger at a particular movement by continually performing that movement. For example, you will get stronger at squats by continually performing squats, over time. This principle holds true for any type of anaerobic or aerobic exercise. Several of the systems I'll talk about use specificity as an advantage to making faster muscular gains by prescribing exercise selection.

# The Variability Principle

The body is exceptionally good at adapting to change, therefore it's beneficial to constantly vary at least one training criteria each time a muscle group is exercised in order to continue the body's adaptation to stress and avoid plateaus. Here, you can see the association between variability and overload— some of the training systems discussed later use this association to great advantage.

That's a good summary of the basic principles of resistance training. Now, let's start our in-depth exploration by looking at one of the earliest weight training systems devised—it's also the most popular.

# Volume Training

Publication of *The Stress of Life*, along with the Weider magazines and the results from early practitioners, such as John Grimek, Clarence Ross and Armand Tanny, ushered in the era of volume training, or High-Volume Training (HVT) in the 1950s. Volume training consists of numerous sets performed for each muscle group, split routines and frequent training sessions—the most common type of training observed in gyms and fitness centers worldwide today. The volume of work subjected to the body is much greater with this type of training than with other systems that emphasize intensity over volume, such as Hardgainer, Heavy Duty, HIT, and SuperSlow.

Formal volume training systems recommend a certain amount of training based on experience level:

- **Beginner**:    Less than one year training
- **Intermediate**:    1-2 years of training
- **Advanced**:    3 or more years of training

The table below presents typical amounts of work recommended for each muscle group, based on those experience levels. (Note: these are working sets and do not include warm-up sets.)

|  | Beginner | Intermediate | Advanced |
|---|---|---|---|
| Abs | 3 | 4-5 | 6-7 |
| Back | 4-5 | 6-8 | 10-12 |
| Biceps | 3-4 | 4-5 | 5-6 |
| Calves | 4 | 5-6 | 6-8 |
| Chest | 4-5 | 6-8 | 10-12 |
| Deltoids | 3-4 | 4-5 | 6-7 |
| Forearms | 2 | 3 | 4 |
| Hamstrings | 2-3 | 3-4 | 5-6 |
| Quadriceps | 4-5 | 6-8 | 10-12 |
| Trapezius | 2-3 | 3-4 | 5-6 |
| Triceps | 4-5 | 5-6 | 6-7 |

# German Volume Training

One specific type of volume training is German Volume Training, popularized in the 1970s by the German National Weightlifting Team and advocated by Vince Gironda in the United States during the 1950s and 1960s.

The goal of German Volume Training is to complete ten sets of ten reps with the same weight on a basic compound movement, with constant rest intervals. Typically, a traditional German Volume Training workout will consist of one or two main exercises, each performed for ten sets of ten reps, along with several other isolation exercises performed for three sets per exercise.

The suggested starting weight for this type of training is 60% of your 1RM in that exercise. For example, if you can squat 300 pounds for one rep, then your starting weight would be 180 pounds for ten reps (300 x 0.6 = 180). Use the same weight on each successive set while maintaining ten reps per set. As the muscle fatigue accumulates as each set is completed, the temptation to take longer rests between sets rises—however, German Volume Training explicitly enforces a constant rest interval between sets, thus increasing the intensity through both the rest interval and increasing loads. In isolation, watching someone perform one or two sets of an exercise at their 60% 1RM level may seem relatively easy—but keep watching—it's the constant, unrelenting pounding that tells the whole story.

Here's an example of a chest workout using the German Volume Training system:

| Exercise | Sets | Reps | Rest |
|---|---|---|---|
| Barbell Bench Press | 10 | 10 | 3 min |
| Incline Dumbbell Press | 3 | 6-8 | 1.5 min |
| Incline Dumbbell Flys | 3 | 10-12 | 1 min |

Here's an example of a leg workout using the German Volume Training system:

| Exercise | Sets | Reps | Rest |
| --- | --- | --- | --- |
| Barbell Squats | 10 | 10 | 3 min |
| Lying Leg Curls | 10 | 10 | 1.5 min |
| Seated Calf Raises | 3 | 15-20 | 1 min |
| Standing Calf Raises | 3 | 12-15 | 1 min |

German Volume Training does not use forced reps, negatives, partials or any of the other typical intensity techniques. However, there is no rule stating that you cannot combine this training system with any other type of intensity technique, as long as your recovery system can handle the increased stress without going into a state of exhaustion (over-training).

Variations of the standard German Volume Training system incorporate differing rep schemes per workout, while continuing with ten sets of the target exercise.

For example, the six-week training routine for chest, listed below, keeps you at 10 sets, but uses differing rep schemes each chest workout in order to increase strength on the bench press:

| Workout | Sets | Reps |
| --- | --- | --- |
| Week 1 | 10 | 8 |
| Week 2 | 10 | 7 |
| Week 3 | 10 | 6 |
| Week 4 | 10 | 5 |
| Week 5 | 10 | 4 |
| Week 6 | 10 | 10 |

Try to increase the weight each week by approximately 5%.

So, the 1950s ushered in the era of volume training, where performing lots of sets for each body part became popular. The next decade would introduce another variation on this approach.

# Peripheral Heart Action (PHA) Training

Chuck Coker, inventor of the *Universal*™ multi-station exercise machines, developed the Peripheral Heart Action (PHA) training system in the early 1960s as a system for developing overall fitness. It's a form of volume training, so get ready to perform lots of sets. The difference here is the minimal rest (if any) between sets, and the ordering of the exercises you select.

The main concept of PHA is to force blood flow up and down the body by working every major muscle group while maintaining an elevated heart rate. This is accomplished by alternating upper body and lower body exercises—as muscles in the upper body are worked, the muscles in the lower body can rest, and vice-versa. The goal of this training system is improved strength, muscle size, cardiovascular efficiency and flexibility. Think of PHA Training as carefully crafted circuit training for your muscles. It's no coincidence that Chuck's *Universal*™ machines were optimized for these types of workouts. Today, many gyms have circuits of machines set up this way, and the Curves™ chain of women's fitness centers include this approach. But don't think it's just for women—PHA Training, done correctly with challenging weights, can be brutal and will definitely improve muscular endurance.

## PHA Training

- Work all major muscle groups in alternating sequences
- Work at a fast pace in order to maintain an elevated heart rate

Typically, PHA training uses a series of sequences, where each sequence consists of a group of exercises to be performed non-stop for a prescribed number of reps. Each sequence is repeated for two or more times, then the next sequence is started. Take rest between sequences only if necessary.

The target heart rate (THR) for PHA training is 220 minus your age, multiplied by 0.8. Accelerate or slow down your training pace, based on your target heart rate.

## PHA Target Heart Rate = (220 - Age) x 0.8

For example, if you are 30 years old, your heart rate should stay around 150 for most of your workout.

Here's some PHA Target Heart Rates (beats per minute) for other ages for quick reference:

| Age | PHA Target Heart Rate |
|-----|-----------------------|
| 20 | 160 |
| 25 | 155 |
| 30 | 150 |
| 35 | 148 |
| 40 | 144 |
| 45 | 140 |
| 50 | 136 |
| 55 | 132 |
| 60 | 128 |

Let's look at a typical PHA training program:

## Sequence 1

- Shoulder Press
- Crunches
- Squats
- Triceps Extensions

## Sequence 2

- Lat Pulldowns
- Hyperextensions
- Lying Leg Curls
- Dumbbell Curls

## Sequence 3

- Bench Press
- Side Bends
- Leg Extensions
- Dips

## Sequence 4

- Bent-over Barbell Rows
- Side Bends
- Standing Calf Raises
- Shrugs

You can set the target number of reps per sequence or per workout depending on your goal(s) for that sequence or training session. For example, you might want to perform your first sequence with higher reps (15-20) to get your heart rate elevated. Then, on the next sequence lower the reps down to 10-12 to keep your heart rate constant. Finally, you can throw in some lower rep sequences (4-8) to build strength and muscle size. Regardless of the reps you choose, make sure your heart rate remains right around that target level—otherwise, you're just doing regular volume training.

Some individuals use PHA Training as a part of their overall Periodization plan, where this type of workout is performed for one week out of an eight week training cycle.

While most people used PHA Training or traditional Volume Training during the 1950s and 1960s, others were formulating a diametrically opposite way to work out. Let's take a look at that next.

# High Intensity Training (HIT)

The High-Intensity Training philosophy was originally developed in the 1960s by Arthur Jones, and later refined and adapted by advocates such as Ellington Darden, Matt Brzycki and Ken Hutchins, among others.

This system of training is a reaction to high volume training, arguing that low volume, coupled with high-intensity is the most effective method to increase both muscle size and strength without over-training. The theory of high-intensity training centers around the dichotomy of working out at either a high-intensity or for a long duration—with the realization that you can't do both at the same time. The classic example is the sprinter versus the distance runner. The sprinter is engaging in a high-intensity activity; however, since he cannot physically maintain the intensity of that activity, it's relatively short in duration. Conversely, the distance runner is working at a much lower intensity and can therefore sustain that level for a much longer duration. The system of high-intensity training carries this example from the aerobic world to the anaerobic world of weight training. HIT advocates want you to visualize and contrast the body types of the low-intensity distance runner with that of the high-intensity sprinter. Which has more muscle?

The original HIT tenet from Jones was the performance of a single, high-intensity set to failure for each muscle group. To support this tenet, Jones led the Colorado Experiment, where professional bodybuilder Casey Viator gained 63 pounds of muscle in only 28 days. Although the experiment was only ever conducted on two individuals who were both regaining previous muscle mass, the results helped propel the HIT methodology into the mainstream of bodybuilding. Over the decades, the performance of the single high-intensity set has been expanded to allow up to three high-intensity sets per muscle group.

HIT training is in direct contrast to volume training, where performance of multiple sets of each exercise is the norm, with many of those sets at sub-maximal effort. HIT training is also in direct contrast to high-speed, explosive training systems discussed later in this book.

## High Intensity Training

- Short workouts
- 1-3 sets per muscle group
- Perform each set to muscular failure
- Work muscles from largest to smallest
- Use good form
- Work out 2-3 times per week

Traditionally, the medical community has thought of resistance training as a poor method for improving cardiovascular fitness. However, high-intensity resistance training offers significant cardiovascular benefits, due to the increased stimulus on the cardiovascular system (this is the only similarity here with PHA Training). In any form of weight training, the greater the cardiovascular stimulus, the more profound the cardiovascular adaptation on the body.

Matt Brzycki, former Princeton University strength coach, developed Ten Commandments of the High Intensity Training philosophy (reflecting the almost religious zealot-like following of this training philosophy):

1. Train with a high level of intensity.
2. Attempt to increase the resistance used or the repetitions performed every workout.
3. Perform 1 to 3 sets of each exercise.
4. Reach muscular failure within a prescribed number of repetitions.
5. Perform each repetition with proper technique.
6. Strength train for no more than one hour per workout.
7. Emphasize the major muscle groups.
8. Whenever possible, work your muscles from largest to smallest.
9. Strength train 2 to 3 times per week on non-consecutive days.
10. Keep accurate records of your performance.

Let's look at each of these HIT Commandments in more detail.

## Train with a High Level of Intensity

Typically, in weightlifting the definition of a high-level of intensity is performing an exercise to the point of concentric muscular failure (lifting the weight). The HIT system also includes the concept of post-fatigue repetitions, beyond concentric failure, by performing additional repetitions via various intensity-boosting techniques, such as negatives, rest/pause, drop sets, etc. HIT argues that failure to reach an appropriate level of intensity will result in little to no gain in strength or muscular size. In other words, with HIT training, you always lift to failure. Notice also that this is in direct conflict with the GAS principle, which calls for periods of high-intensity training, followed by periods of lower-intensity, in order for compensation and growth to occur.

## Attempt to Increase the Resistance Used or the Repetitions Performed Every Workout

This is also known as the single/double progression technique (resistance/repetitions). Notice that this HIT Commandment is in direct conflict with the GAS principle as well, since you attempt increases in reps or weight *every workout*.

## Perform 1 To 3 Sets of Each Exercise

Here, genetics will largely dictate the number of sets to perform—individuals with predominantly white, fast-twitch fibers will generally require fewer sets than individuals with predominantly red, slow-twitch fibers, due to inherent recovery ability. This also holds true for the number of reps and the number of workouts per week. So, how do you know which fiber type is dominant in your body or in certain muscle groups within your body? Try high-volume training for 6-8 weeks, then switch to high-intensity training for 6-8 weeks and note the results to your physique. Repeat this several times, if necessary. Over time, you'll learn how many sets and reps you need for each body part in order to get the results you want. Joe Weider named this technique the Instinctive Training Principle.

## Reach Muscular Failure within a Prescribed Number of Reps

In general, the HIT system prescribes differing rep ranges for different areas of the body:

- Lower Body  (10-15 reps)
- Upper Body  (6-12 reps)

Use the same technique as above to determine how many reps each of your muscle groups responds to best.

## Perform Each Repetition with Proper Technique

The HIT system uses the concept of a "quality rep", which is defined as the raising and lowering of the weight in a deliberate, controlled manner. Quality reps should take approximately 1-2 seconds to lift the weight, and 3-4 seconds to lower the weight. Thus, quality reps are based on exercise form and rep speed. HIT does not advise lifting weights in rapid or explosive fashion, due to the exposure of the muscles, joints and connective tissues to extreme forces, and due to the introduction of momentum during speed training. Prescription of rep speed is explicitly described in order to minimize this momentum. Notice that the SuperSlow system, a type of high-intensity training, virtually eliminates momentum as its central tenet.

## Strength Train for No More Than One Hour per Workout

This is based on the intensity/volume tradeoff, where if you are training with a high-enough level of intensity, you should not be able to sustain that intensity level for more than one hour (remember the sprinter?). In the HIT system, the theory is you can train hard—but not for long, so make the most of it.

## Emphasize the Major Muscle Groups

Since the intensity level of the workout must be high, you should work the major muscle groups (e.g., legs, back, and chest) first in order to maximize muscular gain. If you have a specific body part weakness, and this weakness is with a minor muscle group, such as the biceps, then the HIT system still advocates emphasizing the major muscle groups first, rather than prioritizing your training around the weakness. So, you guys that like to do biceps for an hour might want to wise up and reconsider.

## Whenever Possible, Work Your Muscles from Largest to Smallest

This HIT commandment goes hand-in-hand with the previous one, since the major muscle groups are also the largest. In this system, the recommended order to work your muscles is:

1. Legs (quadriceps, hamstrings, calves)
2. Chest
3. Back
4. Shoulders
5. Biceps
6. Triceps
7. Forearms
8. Abdominals
9. Low Back

(Astute readers will notice that this ordering is not strictly from largest to smallest muscle group—HIT balances this with the push/pull technique, where you alternate working muscle groups for pushing, with those that pull. That's why in the ordering of Shoulders > Biceps > Triceps above, the triceps appear after biceps, even though the triceps muscle complex is much larger than the biceps. Here, you push with the shoulders, pull with the biceps, then push with the triceps.)

Notice that the core muscles are worked last. Advocates of core training would disagree with this approach, but HIT devotees (disciples?) argue that if you are working quads, back, and shoulders with squats, deadlifts and standing overhead presses, your core is getting one hell of a workout throughout. Also, notice that the most popular muscles trained in gyms everywhere—chest and biceps—are listed second and fifth in the HIT prioritization order.

## Strength Train 2 to 3 Times per Week on Non-Consecutive Days

This commandment centers on the body's recovery ability, where it typically requires 48 to 72 hours for muscle tissue to repair itself from a workout. It's also trying to avoid Selye's Exhaustion Stage in the GAS principle. The following variables dictate whether to train two versus three times per week:

- **Larger muscles** (legs, chest, and back) take longer (72 hours) to recover than smaller ones.

- **Age**—the older you get, the longer it takes to recover.

- **Progress**—in this system, as long as you are realizing at least single progression (reps or weight) gains, then your recovery ability is able to keep pace with the exercise demands.

Therefore, older weightlifters who work large muscle groups would probably only work out two times per week under this system and younger lifters performing the same workout could go three times per week.

Notice that most traditional split-systems and programs such as The Bulgarian Method, which advocate working out multiple times per day almost every day of the week, are in direct opposition of this HIT commandment.

## Keep Accurate Records of Your Performance

Training records become a barometer of accomplishment and a roadmap for further progress. This is true under any of the resistance training systems in this book. In HIT, the records form the basis for increasing workout intensity.

Ellington Darden espoused twelve High Intensity Training Guidelines to complement Brzycki's commandments:

1. Perform no more than 20 total sets in any one training session.

2. Train no more than three times a week. Each workout should involve the entire body, as opposed to splitting the routine into lower and upper body workouts on separate days.

3. Select resistance for each exercise that allows you to perform 8-12 reps. Use 15-20 rep for the lower body.

4. Continue each exercise to momentary muscular failure. When you can perform more than the recommended number of repetitions, increase the resistance by approximately 5 percent at the next workout.

5. Work your largest muscles first and your smallest muscles last.

6. Accentuate the negative or lowering portion of each rep. Lift the weight in two seconds and lower it in four seconds.

7. Move slower, never faster, if in doubt about the speed of movement.

8. Attempt to constantly increase the number of reps or the amount of weight—but do not sacrifice form in an attempt to increase reps or weight.

9. Get plenty of rest after each training session. High-intensity exercise necessitates a recovery period of at least 48 hours. Muscles grow during rest, not during exercise.

10. Eat a balanced diet composed of several servings a day from the four basic food groups (fruit and vegetables, dairy, meat, grains). Protein supplements and vitamin-mineral pills are not necessary.

11. Train with a partner who can reinforce proper form on each exercise.

12. Keep accurate records—date, order of exercises, resistance, reps, and overall training time—of each workout.

Using these guidelines, Darden prescribes a typical workout:

| Exercise | Reps |
| --- | --- |
| 1. Squat | 20 |
| 2. Straight-arm Pullover w/Dumbbell | 12 |
| 3. Squat | 20 |
| 4. Straight-arm Pullover w/Dumbbell | 12 |
| 5. Leg Extension | 12 |
| 6. Leg Curl | 12 |
| 7. One-Leg Calf Raise | 15 |
| 8. One-Leg Calf Raise | 15 |
| 9. Press Behind Neck | 12 |
| 10. Chin-Up (behind neck) | 12 |
| 11. Bench Press | 12 |
| 12. Bent-over Row | 12 |
| 13. Dips | 12 |
| 14. Biceps Curl | 12 |
| 15. Triceps Extension w/Dumbbell | 12 |
| 16. Chin-Up (to front) | 12 |
| 17. Dips | 12 |
| 18. Stiff-Legged Deadlift | |
| 19. Wrist Curls | 12 |
| 20. Crunches | 12 |

Note that most HIT workouts are constructed around whole-body routines, due to the intensity, brevity and need for recuperation. As Arthur Jones continually emphasized, "Split routines make about as much sense as sleeping with one eye open."

Darden also noted that as you age, high-intensity training typically places slightly more emphasis on form, rather than pure intensity at the expense of form. Younger bodies (15-40 yrs.) handle cheating better, and recover more quickly from relaxation of form and occasional cheating exercises, than older bodies.

Finally, Darden's adaptation of high-intensity training also incorporates Not-to-Failure (NTF) workout sessions occasionally during the training cycle. These NTF sessions instruct the weightlifter to use their regular training poundage, but to stop two reps short of positive failure (or the previous best effort) on each set. The purpose of the NTF sessions is to aid the body's recovery ability during a schedule of normal HIT training. Perhaps this was Darden's acquiescence that the increasingly popular Periodization concept was useful and could work well within the HIT framework.

# Periodization

Although periodization training has been around since the ancient Greeks prepared for the Olympic Games, Soviet sport scientist Dmitri Matveyev first formalized the general training concept of periodization (cycle training) in the 1960s, as a method for mapping out the entire year's training program through periods of maximal and submaximal work (intensity). This method is based on the results of scientific research on how best to develop an athlete to his/her fullest potential. The rationale behind periodization is that you cannot train the same way all the time. To do so will cause stagnation and plateaus in strength, muscle mass, speed and explosiveness. By performing different types of work over a period of time you can make steady progress, achieving peak performance, conditioning and muscular development at specified times. Of all the training systems, periodization requires the most planning. Additionally, it's advised that you accompany each cycle with specific supplementation, diet, and recovery plans in addition to the training plan.

For periodization discussions in this section, I will focus solely on periodization as applied to bodybuilding training—the purpose here being building maximum muscle size and avoiding plateaus, injury and overtraining.

A "period" refers to the entire length of the training cycle, typically one year, commonly divided into multiple training cycles:

- **Macrocycle**: the entire training cycle (typically one year)

- **Mesocycles**: specific training cycles within the macrocycle, *devoted to a specific purpose*, such as strength/power, mass, or definition. Typically, these cycles last from 6-8 weeks but can be longer or shorter, as we'll see.

- **Microcycle**: specific training variation within the mesocycle, typically varying the training intensity from day to day.

The whole key to periodization is to plan what you are going to change—volume, intensity, exercise selection, rep speed, rest intervals, etc. This helps alleviate boredom and keeps the body adapting. Just keeping yourself interested and motivated to train over a long period of time is the often the biggest hurdle and one of the biggest factors for success in building sustainable muscle.

## Periodization = Planning

Which is why periodization doesn't work for most—by nature, people aren't planners. You have to train yourself to plan out your workouts in order to reach your goals. Additionally, periodization isn't magic—you can't out-periodize your genetics, drug users, or stupidity. But intelligence, smart training and persistence can. Just ask lifetime drug-free bodybuilder and 5-time Mr. Universe Skip La Cour.

Training to failure is not part of the periodization system (the focus is on success—not failure). Ed Coan was a big proponent of this concept. Considered by some the greatest powerlifter in history, he thought it was vitally important to end each workout with a success—for both physical and mental reasons. Only during the actual competition would failure occur—hopefully, after you have achieved a personal best lift or all-time best level of muscularity and conditioning.

There are two general types of periodization—Classic (Linear) and Modern (Non-Linear).

# Classic (Linear) Periodization

This is type of periodization that Matveyev first formalized. It's linear, since you complete each mesocycle in a specific order, progressing from one to the other.

At its simplest, a classic, linear bodybuilding periodization scheme has three cycles or phases:

### PHASE I: Bulking and Mass Building

The goal here is to build more muscle size. This phase is typified by the use of extremely heavy weights, straight sets with looser form and longer rest periods. Interestingly, this is how you see most men training in gyms today—except they do it year round.

## PHASE II: Cutting and Leaning Out

The goal here is to maintain the muscle mass you built in Phase I while reducing your body fat. This phase if typified by the use of moderate weights, supersets and compound sets, more volume, more variety of exercises, higher reps, shorter rest periods and the use of some exercise machines in addition to free weights.

## PHASE III: Active Rest and Recovery

The goal here is to maintain the muscle mass and body fat level you achieved during the first two phases, while giving the body some additional rest, in preparation for the next cycle.

This is the type of periodization many bodybuilders from the 1950s through the 1970s used (the infamous "bulking up and cutting" process). It's how Arnold trained to win all those Mr. Universe and Mr. Olympia titles (the movie *Pumping Iron* famously depicted Arnold training with Phase II style, and then after his victory, starting Phase III by smoking a joint). Other versions of linear periodization routines include Hypertrophy Specific Training (HST), where you progress in two-week cycles from sets of 15 reps, to sets of 10, 8, 5, followed by negative reps—then take a week off and repeat. *Ironman* magazine has long recommended an 8-week linear periodization training regime like this, where you train at full intensity for six weeks, then back off for the final two weeks, before repeating. Doggcrapp (DC) training is almost exactly the same, except it uses the terms "blasts" and "cruises" for the six and two week periods.

# Modern Periodization

Shortly after Matveyev formalized the linear method of periodization, others such as Westside Barbell's powerlifting guru Louie Simmons developed and promoted other periodization methods, including non-linear, undulating and conjugate versions.

These modern versions use much shorter mesocycles, typically 1-2 week training blocks, in order to preserve as much of the results of each cycle into the following period.

Strict non-linear periodization uses straight 1-2 week mesocycles, typically varying (undulating) the rep ranges:

- **Weeks 1-2:** 10-12 reps
- **Weeks 3-4:** 5-6 reps
- **Weeks 4-5**: 7-9 reps
- **Weeks 6-7:** 3-5 reps

You can see from the sample undulating periodization routine above, cycles of higher, then lower reps are alternated, in order to preserve both strength and size gains throughout.

Modern periodization, as applied to bodybuilding, typically contains four phases:

## PHASE I: Strength & Power

- Exclusively compound exercises
- Weights should be about 85% of your 1RM
- 1-5 reps per set
- Lift explosively
- 3-5 minutes rest between sets

## PHASE II: Power Bodybuilding

- Predominantly compound exercises
- Weights should be about 80-85% of your 1RM
- 4-6 reps per set
- Lift quickly
- 3 minutes rest between sets

## PHASE III: Traditional Bodybuilding

- Mix of compound and isolation exercises
- Weights should be about 70-80% of your 1RM
- 8-12 reps per set
- Lift with a moderate tempo (2 seconds up, 3 down)
- 1-2 minutes rest between sets

# PHASE IV: Active Rest (Transition)

- Take one week off from weight training and go walking, hiking, etc.
- Allow your body to rest, recover and transition into the next cycle.

With this type of modern periodized bodybuilding approach, you set the length of each phase, although two week phases are common.

Originally developed in Russia by Dr. Yuri Verkhoshansky, conjugate periodization shortens the length of each mesocycle down to a single week. This is the modern form of periodization that Louie Simmons has successfully used to build some of the largest of most powerful physiques in America over the past several decades. All rep ranges are trained during the week in order to maximize strength, power, size and muscular endurance.

For example, if you train on a 3-day per week schedule, here's how you might structure your workouts with conjugate periodization:

**Day 1**: 3-5 reps
**Day 2**: 8-10 reps
**Day 3**: 10-15 reps

For those who use split-routines and work specific muscle groups on separate days, you can modify this schedule like this:

**Back—workout A**: 3-5 reps
**Back—workout B**: 8-10 reps
**Back—workout C**: 10-15 reps

As you can see, the main difference between classic and modern periodization is the length of each cycle. While classic periodization measured cycles in months, modern versions shortened that to several weeks and even to a single week. You'll see later how Fred Hatfield took this to another level and advocated a periodization scheme within a single workout—what came to be known as Holistic Training.

Both classic and modern versions of periodization acknowledge that you have to back off your training after a while, in order to allow your body to fully rest and recover. It's one thing to be consistent in your training, but another to be stupid and myopic.

Periodization is a powerful concept and I've only scratched the surface here. I encourage you to check out the writings of Louie Simmons and the Westside Barbell Club for much more on this.

While periodization acknowledges that you can't train the same way all the time, others held diametrically opposite views, as we'll see next.

# The Bulgarian Method

During the 1970s, members of the Bulgarian national weightlifting team were the dominant weightlifters in the world, as evidenced by their consistent top placings at the Olympic Games and World Championships in all weight categories. It turns out, the Bulgarians trained far differently than others (they also used heavy amounts of anabolic steroids). Ivan Abadjiev, head coach of the national team, crafted a training methodology so distinct, so sinister, that outsiders cringed and insiders named him "The Butcher".

Under Abadjiev's Bulgarian Method, weightlifters trained 2-6 times per day, six days per week—not unlike many volume-oriented bodybuilders of the 1960s (twice per day, six days per week). However, there were no assigned "light" days. No off-season. Ever. And they trained for specificity, following Selye's Specificity Principle, performing just a few exercises over and over again. Clearly, the Bulgarians rejected the concept of periodization and embraced the concept of forcing—basically demanding—adaptation, not coaxing it, as previous methods sought.

To Abadjiev, this was the only way to train:

*"When a rabbit is being chased by the wolf, does he have an interim stage for running? Yes, he can hide in the bushes but he is ready to start running one hundred percent at any time. Is it logical to achieve outstanding results by hard work and then to stop and to go back to a lower level?"*

## The Bulgarian Method

- **Train for 2 to 6 sessions per day (frequency)**
- **Use extremely heavy weights all the time (overload)**
- **Concentrate on specific exercises or body parts (specificity)**

The bodybuilding community took the concepts in the Bulgarian Method and quickly adopted them within a periodization system, where the techniques would be applied for short 2-4 week bursts, in order to increase strength rapidly. Additionally, they used this method to bring up lagging muscle groups by overloading them far more frequently than others. Arnold Schwarzenegger describes how he used a variation of the Bulgarian Method in *Education of a Bodybuilder*, in order to bring up his calves and rear delts. Upon rising from sleep, Arnold would reach under his bed for a set of dumbbells he had stashed there, proceeding to perform ten sets of rear laterals every morning. For his stubborn calves, former Mr. Universe Reg Park showed him how to attack them with frequent use of super-heavy loads, performing standing calf raises in excess of 1,000 lbs, in order to force the muscles into adaptive growth.

One important note about the Bulgarian Method is the effect it has on both the mind and body. By forcing the use of extremely heavy loads, the weightlifter learns to confront and defeat their fear of poundages previously thought impossible. This effect and the other concepts in the Bulgarian Method would later reappear in other systems, such as Power Factor Training, Positions of Flexion and Static Contraction Training.

Critics of the Bulgarian Method have argued that the system pushes the body into an over-trained and possibly injured state more readily than most other systems. It's also clearly not for beginners. Keep this in mind.

Since most bodybuilders share common weaknesses with lagging rear delt and hamstring development (ever see a bodybuilder whose rear delts or hamstrings were too big?—I thought not), in comparison to their front delts and quads, here are some example Bulgarian-based workouts to improve those areas.

## Bulgarian-based Rear Delt Workouts

Assuming you don't want to use Arnold's dumbbells under the bed tactic described earlier, here are some things you can do every time you step into the gym.

Rear Delt Machine:              5 sets of 6-8 reps (after warming up)
Bent over Dumbbell Laterals:    5 sets of 6-8 reps (after warming up)

Do one of these exercises first in your workout, every workout you do. To up the ante even further, do them again at the end of your workout.

Here's another variation:

Rear Delt Machine:          1 set of 6-8 reps
Bent over Dumbbell Laterals:   1 set of 6-8 reps

Do one set of either of these exercises between every regular set in your workout, regardless of what muscle group you are currently working. For example, if you are working chest and back that day, perform a set for your chest, then a rear delt set. Then, go back to your chest exercise, followed by a rear delt set. Continue your entire workout this way—by the end of the workout you'll have performed a lot of rear delt work (frequency) with heavy loads (overload) just for that body part (specificity). Do this every workout for a couple weeks, then go back to your normal routine.

## Bulgarian-based Hamstring Workouts

Using the same tactics described above for the rear delts, here's some Bulgarian-based work you can do to improve your hamstrings.

Leg curls (lying, sitting or standing):   5 sets of 6-8 reps (after warm up)
Stiff-Leg Deadlifts:                      5 sets of 6-8 reps (after warm up)

Do one of these exercises first in your workout, every workout you do. To up the ante even further, do them again at the end of your workout. Just make sure that both you and your hamstrings are thoroughly warmed up before attacking them—hamstring injuries typically occur with cold, tight hamstrings. Make sure they are ready to go.

Here's another variation:

Leg curls:          1 set of 6-8 reps
Stiff-Leg Deadlifts:   1 set of 6-8 reps

Do one set of either of these exercises between every regular set in your workout, regardless of what muscle group you are currently working—same as described above.

These workouts should give you ideas for incorporating similar types of routines for whatever muscle group(s) you need to bring up to par with the rest of your physique.

# Pre-Exhaustion Training

Robert Kennedy, former publisher of *MuscleMag International* and other fitness-oriented magazines started advocating the use of pre-exhaustion training in the early 1970s. The concept of pre-exhaustion, where you perform a compound movement immediately following a single-joint isolation movement, was initially pioneered by Arthur Jones and his introduction of High-Intensity Training and Nautilus exercise equipment in the 1960s.

The purpose of pre-exhaustion is to avoid the situation where a smaller assistance muscle fails before the larger, primary muscle reaches complete muscular failure. For example, most guys love to bench press—and most of the time, their smaller, relatively weaker triceps muscles which assist in the press, fail before the pectorals are fully exhausted. In this case, pre-exhaustion training advocates the use of an isolation exercise, such as dumbbell flys, to be used immediately before starting to bench press. This will pre-fatigue (pre-exhaust) the chest, while keeping the triceps at full strength (since they aren't involved in a fly motion). When the bench press is done immediately after the flys are finished, the chest is partially fatigued, the triceps are strong, and chances are your chest will completely fatigue before your triceps do.

The key here is to perform the compound exercise **immediately** after the isolation exercise, with no rest in between. Arthur Jones designed his original Nautilus machines this way—the leg press machine also contained a leg extension unit, the shoulder press machine contained a lateral raise, etc.

## Pre-Exhaustion Training

**Perform an isolation exercise immediately followed by a compound exercise for the same muscle group**

While Kennedy advocated performing entire workouts in pre-exhaustion style, modern variations also use it just for portions of a workout (Weider's Pre-Exhaustion Principle), often performed with chest (fly/press) and quads (extension/squat), although you can employ it with any muscle group. Using our earlier example, a typical pre-exhaust set for chest would have perform dumbbell flys immediately followed by dumbbell presses. As your chest gets tired from the flys, you switch to presses, which now uses your triceps to help you complete each rep. Notice that this is completely opposite of what typically happens when you perform presses for your chest—your triceps tend to tire out before your chest does, right? Pre-Exhaustion throws this in reverse.

The big disadvantage to Pre-Exhaustion training is that you won't be able to use your normal heavier weights on the second exercise, since your target muscle is already fatigued from the isolation movement.

Here are some good Pre-Exhaust exercise combos to try:

| Muscle Group | Pre-Exhaustion Exercise Combos |
|---|---|
| Back | Pullovers + Chins or Pulldowns |
| | Pullovers + Rows |
| Biceps | Concentration Curls + Barbell Curls |
| Chest | Flys + Presses |
| | Flys + Dips |
| Legs | Leg Extensions + Squats or Leg Presses |
| | Leg Curls + Stiff-Leg Deadlifts |
| Traps | Shrugs + Upright Rows |
| Triceps | Pushdowns + Dips |
| | Extensions + Close-Grip Bench Press |

While Arthur Jones pioneered the scientific concept of increasing muscle fatigue through pre-exhaustion training and Kennedy advocated its use through his publications, one of Jones' pupils took the science of high-intensity, pre-exhaustion and muscular adaptation to a whole new level that changed the way many bodybuilders train, even to today.

# Heavy Duty

One of Arthur Jones early students, professional bodybuilder Mike Mentzer, developed the Heavy Duty training system during the 1970s. Heavy Duty incorporates a general scientific philosophy of maximum effort in minimal time, while exhausting a minimum of the body's recuperative abilities. It's essentially pre-exhaustion training, except with minimal sets and maximum intensity applied. You get one shot at each exercise, so make it count.

### Heavy Duty

- Infrequent workouts (two per week)
- Short workouts (30 minutes)
- High intensity (complete eccentric and concentric muscular failure)

Mentzer's Heavy Duty system fundamentally decomposes into seven principles:

1. Identity
2. Intensity
3. Duration
4. Frequency
5. Specificity
6. Adaptation
7. Progression

Let's look at each principle in more detail.

# Principle #1: Identity

This principle forms the foundation the remaining six Heavy Duty principles build upon. Stated simply, identity is the realization and acceptance that weightlifting is a part of exercise science, derived from medical science. As such, all scientific concepts of the body apply to weightlifting: the characteristics, interrelationships, and interactions of muscles, skeletal structures, connective tissue, etc. An example of the principle of identity in practice is the concept of muscle contraction. Since a muscle fiber only contracts completely, there is no concept of partial contraction—either the muscle fiber is contracted or it is not. This black or white, true or false philosophy pervades the Heavy Duty system and depends entirely on it. It's also the principle that uniquely identifies the Heavy Duty system from other High-Intensity systems—this philosophical underpinning.

## Principle #2: Intensity

This principle states that high-intensity muscular contraction is the most important requirement for the stimulation of rapid increases in muscular size and strength. The duration of the exercise is not important for these goals. Consequently, the harder an individual trains, the less time he will be able to train. Therefore, intensity and duration exist in an inverse ratio to each other—you can train hard or you can train long, but you cannot do both (obviously, Mentzer was listening to Jones). In essence, this is the principle by which Mentzer advocated his famously brief training sessions. Mentzer sums up the intensity principle: "The bodybuilder must regularly make the attempt to perform those tasks that seem impossible." Always the philosopher king of bodybuilding, Mentzer channels Nietzsche's famous phrase, "That which does not kill me makes me stronger". (The Bulgarians would agree—but deny the infrequency of training sessions.)

Heavy Duty advocates increasing the intensity of the workout by one (or more) of three methods:

1. **Progressively increasing the weight used.**

2. **Progressively decreasing the amount of time required to perform a workout.**

3. **Performing each set to a point of total muscular failure (both concentric and eccentric failure).**

Mentzer emphasized that the third method of increasing intensity, performing a set to the point of total muscular failure, is the single most important factor in increasing size and strength.

The Heavy Duty system uses several common techniques for increasing intensity and reaching complete muscular failure, including:

- **Forced Reps**
- **Negatives**
- **Partials**
- **Peak Contraction**
- **Pre-Exhaustion**
- **Rest-Pause**
- **Static Contraction**

You'll notice that these borrow from the Weider System, of which Mentzer was an early pupil.

# Principle #3: Duration

The body's limited ability to recover from exercise forms the principle of Duration; therefore, the duration of a workout, measured by the volume of sets performed, becomes a negative factor in recovery. For every set performed, the body will require more time to recover. Based on this, Mentzer advocated that optimal results from weightlifting are achieved by performing only the minimal volume of sets in order to induce muscular change. Since Mentzer's Intensity Principle tells us that muscular growth is stimulated through high-intensity training and since the higher the intensity of a workout the shorter the duration of the workout, a high-intensity workout must be low volume. Typical Heavy Duty workout sessions last no longer than thirty minutes.

# Principle #4: Frequency

There is a strong relationship between the principles of Frequency and Duration, in that both relate to the body's ability to recover from exercise. While Duration is concerned with the amount of work performed during a single workout, Frequency is concerned with how many workouts are performed during a given time period, such as a week or month. Heavy Duty advocates performing the least number of workouts per week while stimulating muscular growth, in order to maximize the body's ability to recover and elicit this growth. Typical Heavy Duty workout schedules have individuals averaging two workouts per week.

# Principle #5: Specificity

The principle of Specificity recognizes that the developments of certain physical and physiological characteristics are a result of specific forms of exercise. For example, in order to produce large muscles, individuals must typically train with heavy weights using bodybuilding and/or powerlifting exercises. Conversely, you must perform frequent cardiovascular exercise to increase aerobic capacity and increase lung volume. You'll remember from earlier that this principle is not unique to Heavy Duty; Selye's general principle of Specificity is recognized by all weight training systems, as well as in most forms of athletic training.

Besides using bodybuilding/powerlifting exercises to stimulate muscle growth, Heavy Duty tells us that every set of each exercise needs to stimulate the maximum amount of muscle fibers for optimal results. The system prescribes four techniques in order to maximize muscle stimulation during a set:

1. **Start from a Pre-Stretched Position**
   This sets up the myotatic (stretch) reflex and allows for maximum contraction.

2. **Use a Slow Rate of Speed**
   This technique is very similar to the SuperSlow training system philosophy of repetition performance and attempts to eliminate momentum at the beginning of the rep. Slow, deliberate reps reduce damage and wear on connective tissue.

3. **Use a Complete Range of Motion**
   Move the joint through a position of full extension to full contraction. (This differs from other systems, such as Power Factor and Static Contraction.)

4. **Heavy Weights Must Be Used**
   You must use sufficient resistance in order to require a muscle to contract maximally (e.g., firing maximum fibers). Only the exact number of muscle fibers will be recruited to complete the effort—therefore, maximal resistance recruits maximal fibers.

# Principle #6: Adaptation

All of the previous Heavy Duty principles lead to the Principle of Adaptation. Building muscle is the result of the body's adaptation to the stress of infrequent, short-duration, high-intensity exercise. Therefore, the purpose of the principles of Intensity, Duration, Frequency, and Specificity are to cause the principle of Adaptation to occur. Note that this Heavy Duty principle is exactly the same as Selye's General Adaptation Syndrome principle described earlier.

# Principle #7: Progression

The principle of Progression occurs naturally only when the previous six principles are learned (Identity), applied (Intensity, Duration, Frequency, Specificity) and have occurred (Adaptation). When the first six principles are executed consistently, then physical progress should be a constant, predictable occurrence. If you aren't progressing, then your body has adapted to your training intensity—therefore, you must increase the intensity in order for the cycle to begin anew.

Based on the core principles of Intensity, Duration, and Frequency, Mentzer related that individuals who are not progressing in muscular strength and size are due to two probable causes:

1. The intensity of the workouts were not high enough to stimulate the Adaptation response.

2. The workouts were too long and/or the frequency between workouts was too short for adaptation to occur.

If you need to increase the intensity of your workout, Heavy Duty borrows from and recommends the following Weider Training System principles:

- Pre-Exhaustion
- Rest-Pause
- Forced Reps
- Retro-Gravity Reps (Negatives)

Typically, in a Heavy Duty workout you add in each intensity booster in the order listed above, as required. For example, to increase the intensity of a set of the standard barbell bench press you would start with a set of flys (pre-exhaust), then move immediately to the press—pressing until you can't perform another rep. Then, use the Rest-Pause technique until you can't perform another rep in that fashion, at which time have a training partner assist you with some forced reps. When you can't get any more forced reps you can perform some negatives until you can't control the descent of the weight (hopefully, you have a good, trustworthy training partner). That's one set—and your only set under the Heavy Duty model. This is brutally tough training, both mentally and physically.

## Sample Workouts

This section presents some sample Heavy Duty workouts, organized by muscle group.

Note that you should perform all exercises listed as pre-exhaust exercises with the exercise that follows. Additionally, perform all warm-ups with the compound exercise—not the pre-exhaust exercise. Use the four intensity boosting techniques listed earlier as necessary, and appropriate.

| Abdominals | |
|---|---|
| Crunches or Hanging Leg Raises | 1 x 12-20 reps |

| Biceps | |
|---|---|
| General biceps warm-up | 1-3 sets |
| Close-grip, palms-up Pulldowns or Curls (barbell/preacher/machine) | 1 x 6-10 reps |

| Chest | |
|---|---|
| General chest warm-up | 1-3 sets |
| Dumbbell flys or cable crossovers (pre-exhaust) | 1 x 6-10 reps |
| Barbell presses (incline or flat) or Dips | 1 x 1-3 reps |

| Legs | |
|---|---|
| General leg warm-up | 1-3 sets |
| Leg extensions (pre-exhaust) | 1 x 12-20 reps |
| Leg Presses or Squats | 1 x 12-20 reps |
| Calf Raises (standing or donkey) | 1 x 12-20 reps |

| Shoulders | |
|---|---|
| General shoulder warm-up | 1-3 sets |
| Lateral raises (dumbbells or machine) | 1 x 6-10 reps |
| Bent-over laterals (dumbbells or cable) | 1 x 6-10 reps |
| Presses (barbell or machine) or Upright Rows | 1 x 6-10 reps |

| Triceps | |
|---|---|
| General triceps warm-up | 1-3 sets |
| Pushdowns (pre-exhaus) or Lying Extensions | 1 x 6-10 reps |
| Dips or Close-Grip Bench Presses | 1 x 3-5 reps |

If your progress stalls using the workout programs presented above, then Heavy Duty advocates a complete week or two of rest, followed by a short period of Consolidated Workouts. These Consolidated Workouts are extremely brief and intense, thus maximizing your recovery ability.

Here are some samples of Consolidated Workouts:

| Consolidated Workout #1 | |
|---|---|
| Squats or Leg Presses | 1 x 12-20 reps |
| Close-grip, palms-up Pulldowns | 1 x 6-10 reps |
| Dips | 1 x 6-10 reps |

| Consolidated Workout #2 | |
| --- | --- |
| Deadlifts or Shrugs | 1 x 6-10 reps |
| Press Behind Neck | 1 x 6-10 reps |
| Standing Calf Raises | 1 x 12-20 reps |

Although Mentzer advertised his use of Heavy Duty training as the key to his success in professional bodybuilding, he often used periodization, alternating times of Heavy Duty training with periods of more traditional lower-intensity, volume training. In this way, Mentzer and Heavy Duty became a confluence in the late 1970s merging training ideas from the past and guiding them into the future.

# The Weider System

Joe Weider started developing his Weider System of Bodybuilding in 1936. As the decades passed, and the variety of weight training methods emerged, Weider selected the salient points from each, adding them to his meta-system and marketing the concepts (calling them 'principles') with unique names, such as The Retro-Gravity Principle (what we call 'negatives'). It's arguably the most popular system in use today, due to the consistent popularity of Weider's magazines through the decades, starting with *Your Physique* and *Muscle Builder* in the 1950s through the 1970s and continuing with *Muscle & Fitness* and *Flex* today, which serve as monthly reinforcements of "his" principles—not to mention the pictures. The culmination of these principles first appeared with the publication of *The Weider System of Bodybuilding* in 1981.

The Weider System is actually a guide, categorized as 32 training methods/principles, which an individual uses to develop his/her personalized system, based on their unique recuperative abilities, experience, goals, strengths and weaknesses. The guidelines are organized into three broad categories:

1. **Principles for Planning Your Workouts (Cycle-to-Cycle)**
2. **Principles for Arranging Your Workout (Day-to-Day)**
3. **Principles for Performing Each Exercise (Set-to-Set)**

The list of principles is extremely wide-ranging and flexible, since the concepts are pulled from a wide variety of weight training methods. Within each principle are guidelines to assist you in determining whether to use it and the frequency you should use it. But make no mistake about the Weider System—it's a clear advocate of volume training, as if HIT and Heavy Duty never existed.

Here's the complete list of Weider Principles, organized by the three broad categories. Some principles are listed under multiple categories, since they encompass both cycle-to-cycle, and day-to-day methods, or day-to-day and set-to-set methods. One principle, the Instinctive Training Principle appears in all three categories, since it is applicable to all aspects of training.

## Planning Workouts

- Progressive Overload
- Cycle Training
- Split System Training
- Muscle Confusion
- Holistic Training
- Eclectic Training
- Instinctive Training

## Arranging Workouts

- Set System Training
- Superset Training
- Compound Sets Training
- Tri-Sets Training
- Giant Sets Training
- Staggered Sets Training
- Rest-Pause Training
- Muscle Priority Training
- Pre-Exhaustion Training
- Pyramid Training
- Descending Sets Training
- Instinctive Training

## Performing Each Exercise

- Isolation
- Quality Training
- Cheating
- Continuous Tension
- Forced Reps
- Flushing Training
- Burns
- Partial Reps
- Retro-Gravity
- Peak Contraction
- Superspeed
- Iso-Tension
- Instinctive Training

Additionally, the Weider Principles are grouped by experience level for Beginners, Intermediates, and Advanced trainers:

## Beginner (less than 6 months training)

- Progressive Overload
- Set System Training
- Isolation
- Muscle Confusion

## Intermediate (6 months—2 years training)

- Muscle Priority
- Pyramid Training
- Split System Training
- Flushing Training
- Superset Training
- Compound Sets
- Holistic Training
- Cycle Training
- Iso-Tension

## Advanced (more than 2 years training)

- Staggered Sets
- Rest-Pause
- Descending Sets
- Quality Training
- Cheating
- Tri-Sets
- Giant Sets
- Eclectic Training
- Pre-Exhaustion
- Continuous Tension
- Forced Reps
- Burns
- Partial Reps
- Retro-Gravity
- Peak Contraction
- Superspeed
- Instinctive Training

Now that you've seen how each Weider Principle is categorized, let's look at each one in detail and discuss the origins of each.

# Principles for Planning Your Workouts

## Progressive Overload Principle

This is the basic tenet of resistance training codified by Selye. Increase the weight, reps, volume, or intensity of the exercise and training session(s) to overload the muscles.

## Cycle Training Principle

Dividing your training year into cycles for strength, mass, contest preparation, etc., which helps to avoid injuries and keep the body responsive to adaptation. This is periodization.

## Split System Training Principle

This technique has you dividing your workout week into separate training sessions, each targeting specific muscle groups, such as a lower body day, upper body day, a day for chest/triceps, etc. The purpose is to increase the intensity of each training session since you have fewer muscle groups to work and can deliver more concentrated overload to them. Some common split systems include:

- Upper Body/Lower Body (2-Way Split)
- Push/Pull
- Push/Push
- 3-Way Split
- 4-Way Split
- 1 Body Part Per Day

Let's take a look at some examples of these split systems from *The Weider System of Bodybuilding*.

## Weider 2-Way Split

This routine has you work each muscle group twice per week, divided into upper body and lower body.

| MONDAY/THURSDAY | TUESDAY/FRIDAY |
| --- | --- |
| Chest | Back |
| Shoulders | Quads |
| Biceps | Hamstrings |
| Triceps | Forearms |
| Calves | Calves |
| Abs | Abs |

You'll notice that both calves and abs are worked with both upper and lower body, hitting these muscles four times per week. Clearly, Joe thought these areas demanded more work than others.

## Weider 3-Way Split

This routine has you work each muscle group twice per week, but divides the body into three separate workouts, based around push/push and pull/pull schemes. You're now working out six days per week versus the four days in the previous routine (more volume and frequency).

| MON/THURS | TUES/FRI | WED/SAT |
| --- | --- | --- |
| Abs | Abs | Abs |
| Chest | Upper Back | Quads |
| Shoulders | Biceps | Hamstrings |
| Triceps | Forearms | Lower Back |
| Forearms | Calves | Calves |

Weider also presented a blend of those two workout schemes, using the upper body/lower body division of the 2-Way Split with the frequency and volume of the 3-Way Split. The result was the 6-Day Split, using a push/pull scheme.

## Weider 6-Day, 2-Way Split

| MON/WED/FRI | TUES/THUR/SAT |
|---|---|
| Abs | Abs |
| Chest | Quads |
| Shoulders | Hamstrings |
| Upper Back | Lower Back |
| Forearms | Biceps & Triceps |
| Calves | Forearms |
| | Calves |

# Double/Triple Split Training Principle

Divide your workout into two or three shorter, more intense training sessions per day. Here we are getting a variation of The Bulgarian Method.

*The Weider System of Bodybuilding* provides a suggested double-split workout that we can examine:

## Weider Double-Split Workout

| MON/WED/FRI (morning) | TUES/THUR/SAT (morning) |
|---|---|
| ▪ Abs <br> ▪ Chest <br> ▪ Shoulders | ▪ Abs <br> ▪ Quads <br> ▪ Hamstrings <br> ▪ Forearms |

| MON/WED/FRI (evening) | TUES/THUR/SAT (evening) |
|---|---|
| ▪ Calves <br> ▪ Upper Back <br> ▪ Biceps | ▪ Calves <br> ▪ Lower Back <br> ▪ Triceps |

One issue with this type of workout is that on some days (MON/WED/FRI) you are working large muscles in both the morning and evening sessions (chest and back). That's taxing on your recovery system (remember Selye's Exhaustion Stage?). Given Weider's Muscle Priority Principle, where he advocates working larger muscle groups first, he proceeded to produce a variation of this workout that eliminated this problem.

## Weider Double-Split Workout (Muscle Priority version)

| MON/WED/FRI (morning) | TUES/THUR/SAT (morning OR evening) |
|---|---|
| • Abs<br>• Chest<br>• Back<br>• Calves | • Abs<br>• Quads<br>• Hamstrings<br>• Calves<br>• Forearms |

MON/WED/FRI (evening)

• Abs
• Shoulders
• Arms

Notice that this variation works the chest and back together, in push/pull fashion in the morning, while leaving the relatively less demanding shoulders and arms in the evening. It also acknowledges that leg workouts are demanding and exhausting, deserving a single workout on those days—no doubling up.

The big problem with this type of training is time—unless you are independently wealthy or have no immediate family or friends, most people just don't have the time to work out two times each day. Since Weider made a living surrounded by, writing about and marketing things that showcased professional bodybuilders' physiques, this is no surprise. It's also the complete antithesis of the high-intensity school and all its variations.

## Muscle Confusion Principle

Use variation in exercises, sets, reps, and weight, in order to avoid plateaus, alter the level of stress and (hopefully!) continue the adaptation process.

## Holistic Training Principle

Use a variety of rep/set schemes, intensity and frequency of exercises in order to maximize muscle hypertrophy. Dr. Fred Hatfield expanded upon this with his Holistic Training system in the 1980s.

## Eclectic Training Principle

Combine exercise movements for mass, strength, and isolation into a single workout. Again, this is purely Holistic Training.

## Instinctive Training Principle

Construct an individualized program of cycles, routines, exercises, sets, reps, and intensity levels based on experience for maximum results. The key words here are "construct", and "cycles". That's Periodization training—and there is nothing "instinctive" about it.

# Principles for Arranging Your Workout

## Set System Training Principle

Perform multiple sets of each exercise in order to maximize stress. You'll notice that this is the opposite of Heavy Duty.

## Superset Training Principle

Perform two consecutive exercises for *opposing muscle groups*, with no rest between them. Arnold loved to train this way. His classic workouts consisting of a set of bench presses followed by chins, is a prime example. It's a great way to stretch one muscle group, while contracting the opposing muscle group. Other examples include biceps and triceps, quads and hamstrings, front and rear delts, and abs and lower back.

## Compound Sets Training Principle

Perform two consecutive exercises for the *same muscle group*, with no rest between them. Notice that this is not necessarily the same as Pre-Exhaustion Training or Weider's Pre-Exhaustion Principle, since it doesn't specify performing an isolation exercise before a compound movement. You can perform two compound movements for the same muscle one right after the other. If you haven't tried this, it's tough—just don't expect to use your normal weights on the second compound exercise, since the muscle group will already be fatigued.

## Tri-Sets Training Principle

Perform three consecutive exercises for the same muscle group, with no rest between them. This is particularly well-suited for shoulder work, since the shoulder complex consists of three main parts (front, side, rear). You can perform front, side and rear laterals as a tri-set.

## Giant Sets Training Principle

Perform four or more consecutive exercises for the same muscle group, with no rest between them. This technique is often used in abdominal training.

## Staggered Sets Training Principle

Alternate a set of a specific exercise between each set of your regular workout. (Joe talked about it and Arnold did it—or was it Arnold doing it and Joe writing about it?) This is useful to improve underdeveloped body parts. I talked about this technique previously in The Bulgarian Method.

## Rest-Pause Training Principle

Perform your set to failure (or close to failure), then rest for a few seconds, and then perform additional reps, etc. This increases the intensity of the set and was a favorite of Mentzer's, used throughout his Heavy Duty system.

## Muscle Priority Training Principle

Work your weaker muscle groups first in any given workout, when you have the most energy. Working your larger muscles first in the workout is another example of this principle in practice. This is just smart training and sometimes takes courage and fortitude to plow through since most of us have favorite muscle groups, and they usually aren't our weaker ones. You have to constantly mentally battle through doing what you need to do versus what you want/like to do, while keeping this stuff fun.

## Pre-Exhaustion Principle

Perform an isolation exercise first, immediately followed by a compound movement. Working a single-joint assistive muscle group first, followed by the main multi-joint muscle complex, is an example of this principle in practice. Think flys and presses for chest, extensions and squats/presses for legs, etc. While Joe is talking about this as a portion of your workout, keep in mind it's not exactly the same thing as Pre-Exhaustion Training, where it's your entire workout.

## Pyramid Training Principle

Start a series of sets for a muscle group with higher reps and lighter weight, gradually increasing the weight and lowering the reps per set. This process is called half-pyramid training and is used almost universally everywhere you look. You've done it, the guy next to you is doing it right now, and so is most of the rest of the gym. Since Milo did it, it's the oldest trick in the book. A full pyramid has you increasing the weight/lowering the reps until you reach your target weight, and then reversing the process all the way down. Not as common, with much more volume (you're essentially doubling the number of sets), but worth a try every now and again.

## Descending Sets Principle

Lower the weight from set to set as muscle fatigue increases. Other common terms for this technique are "stripping" or "running the rack". The amount of rest you take between sets is variable. One common variation has you taking little to no rest—this is typically what you see when guys are performing strip sets, typically with dumbbell curls, but it's applicable to almost every exercise. Try it with squats, presses or rows for a quick wake-up call. Try it with calf raises and that burning smell will be your calves on fire.

## Instinctive Training Principle

Construct an individualized program of cycles, routines, exercises, sets, reps, and intensity levels for maximum results. This sounds an awful lot like Periodization, doesn't it? It is. You could call it the Planned Training Principle. Most people don't do it, which may be why they fail.

# Principles for Performing Each Exercise

## Isolation Principle

Perform an exercise which targets as few muscles as possible (ideally a single muscle), in order to maximize the stress applied to it. This minimizes the use of stabilizing and synergist muscles. Isolation exercises are single-joint movements (curls, extensions, shrugs) compared to the pushing and pulling multi-joint exercises.

## Quality Training Principle

Gradually reduce the rest between sets while maintaining (or increasing) the number of reps performed. This increases the intensity of the workout session. You'll remember that PHA Training also emphasized minimization of rest intervals between sets.

## Cheating Training Principle

Use body momentum to coax the weight through the sticking point in order to add additional overload. Apply this technique after you can no longer perform reps in good form. As you'll see later, many training systems advocate the exclusive use of strict form and no momentum, particularly SuperSlow, while others such as Heavy Duty use cheating at the end of a set to increase muscle stress and fatigue.

## Continuous Tension Principle

Perform an exercise with relatively slow, constant tension on the muscle(s). This is best accomplished with cable or machine exercises since they provide constant stress throughout the entire range of motion. Free weights generally do not, unless you are training in SuperSlow style.

## Forced Reps Training Principle

Use a training partner to assist you with the completion of a few reps at the end of a set when you can no longer perform a rep on your own. This increases the overload on the muscles and is one of the central methods used with Heavy Duty.

## Flushing Training Principle

Perform three or more exercises for a muscle group before moving on to train another group. This is how most bodybuilders train, working one part of the body with several exercises before moving on to another muscle group. It's the opposite of PHA Training.

## Burns Training Principle

Perform limited short-range movements at the end of the set, after you can't do another rep through the full range of motion. Larry Scott, the first Mr. Olympia used this to great advantage with preacher curls to help build his amazing biceps. It's also very effective with side lateral raises and hamstring curls. Burns are performed in the stretch portion of the movement (near the start)—one of the three key areas in the Positions of Flexion system I'll talk about later.

## Partial Reps Training Principle

Perform an exercise through only a partial range of motion, typically with a weight that causes maximum stress overload for a particular muscle group. Both Power Factor and Positions of Flexion training are based on this principle. Note that Burns are a type of partial-rep—however, burns are performed after full-range reps, while this principle dictates performance of partial-reps throughout the set.

## Retro-Gravity Principle

Perform an exercise by lowering a weight with about 30-40 percent more weight than you can lift on that exercise. This typically requires a training partner for assistance. The common term for this technique is "negatives" and is the final intensity technique used in the all-out barrage of a complete muscular failure set in the Heavy Duty system.

## Peak Contraction Principle

Hold the weight through maximum muscle contraction for a few seconds at the completion of the movement. This typically increases your muscular density over time. You can often literally feel the difference between a bodybuilder who has learned to consistently squeeze the muscles being worked and those who have not. As Arnold's early girlfriends' noted, it's like tickling a rock. Dave Draper, former Mr. Universe and the Blond Bomber, has always noted that weightlifters don't squeeze their muscles hard enough. Squeeze them are hard as you can at the end of the movement, and then squeeze even harder. Finally, Bill Pearl, 5-time Mr. Universe categorized weight trainers as those who lifted weights and those who threw weights around. He was talking about muscle contraction (and the relinquishing of ego).

Here are some common peak contraction exercises:

| | |
|---|---|
| **Abs** | Crunches |
| | Hanging Leg Raises |
| **Back** | Chins |
| | Pulldowns |
| | Rows |
| | Hyperextensions |
| **Biceps** | Concentration Curls |
| | Spider Curls |
| | Machine Curls |
| **Calves** | Calf Raises |
| | Calf Presses |
| **Chest** | Cable Flys |
| | Machine Flys |
| **Forearms** | Wrist Curls |
| **Hamstrings** | All varieties of leg curls |
| **Quadriceps** | Leg Extensions |
| | Leg Adductions/Abductions |
| **Traps** | Shrugs |
| | Upright Rows |
| **Triceps** | Pushdowns |
| | Kickbacks |

## Superspeed Principle

Perform an exercise using acceleration of the movement (e.g. doing the exercise as fast as possible when lifting the weight). This builds explosive muscular power as well as muscle mass. Dr. Fred Hatfield and Lee Haney, 8-time Mr. Olympia, both recognized that some exercises need to be performed explosively and others rhythmically with a tempo. If you always lift a weight using the same rep speed, you'll typically hit a plateau, due to lack of muscular power. Try bench pressing 135lbs explosively—and then with a slower, rhythmic movement. There's a big difference. You won't build up to a big bench or big anything with slower rep tempos. That's the point of this principle. (And it's the complete antithesis of SuperSlow.)

## Iso-Tension Principle

Tense a muscle or muscle group as hard as possible for 5-10 seconds for up to 50 times. This is useful right after you complete a set and can be used with any muscle group, not just your biceps. Again, it builds up your muscle density and is the basis for Static Contraction Training, which I'll discuss shortly.

## Instinctive Training Principle

Use experience to construct an individualized program of cycles, routines, exercises, sets, reps, and intensity levels for maximum results. We've gone over this one twice before.

# The Hardgainer Method

Stuart McRobert developed and popularized the Hardgainer Method during the 1980s in his *Hardgainer* magazine and *Brawn* book series. He defines a "hardgainer" as an individual of average genetic makeup who cannot gain size or strength using volume-training methods. His estimates of the general population who fit this description are 60%-90% of all weight trainers. If you look around your local gym, I think you'll concur.

By McRobert's definition, hardgainers have much less tolerance to exercise than easy gainers and reach an over-trained state much more quickly than others—therefore his methodology calls for performing fewer exercises and sets, and training less frequently but with higher intensity, much like HIT and Heavy Duty.

Individuals using this program should train 2-3 times per week, unless feeling tired. In this case, the philosophy is "when in doubt do less, not more", which is just the opposite of the "if this works, then more should work better" philosophy commonplace in most gyms, as applied to training, supplements, and—dare we say, drugs.

## The Hardgainer Method

- Fewer exercises
- Fewer sets
- Low frequency
- High intensity (train to failure)
- "When in doubt, do less, not more"

The core of the Hardgainer Method consists of basic exercises performed for low sets and high intensity, coupled with intensity cycling (periodization).

Typically, the intensity cycling should follow a pattern of 6-12 weeks of high intensity, followed by four weeks of low intensity. Note that the Hardgainer intensity cycling pattern differs from pure Periodization training, since the Hardgainer Method dictates the use of the same rep scheme throughout and across the cycle, whereas Periodization uses varied rep schemes both during and across cycles.

Here, the general number of reps performed dictates the number of sets to complete. Since the program suggests you use the number of reps that your individualized body most benefits from, some Hardgainers will be using high reps, while others will use moderate or low reps, typically on a muscle group by muscle group basis.

Additionally, the Hardgainer guidelines specify the maximum number of working sets to perform based on the rep ranges used:

- **Low/Moderate Reps (4-10):**     **8 working sets**
- **High Reps (12+):**     **10 working sets**

Based on these guidelines, the Hardgainer Method prescribes no more than 16-30 work sets **per week**. Typically, this is what most volume trainers perform during a single workout.

As mentioned previously, the Hardgainer Method prescribes the use of intensity cycling, which involves several weeks using lighter weights (80%-95% of your typical poundage) without going to positive muscular failure, followed by a few weeks of heavy weights lifted to failure.

As mentioned previously, the emphasis is on basic, compound exercises over isolation exercises.

**The Hardgainer basic exercises include:**

- **Squats**
- **Bench Presses**
- **Overhead Presses**
- **Deadlifts**
- **Rows**
- **Pull-ups**
- **Dips**

Additionally, the Hardgainer Method does not advocate the use of free weights over machines or vice versa—it's exercise-agnostic in this regard. The only stipulation is to use what works best for you, given your structure, injuries, etc. However, there are several exercises which should be avoided, due to the higher injury potential.

**Exercises to avoid include:**

- **Good Mornings**   (low back injury potential)
- **Upright Rows**   (shoulder impingement injury potential)

In general, minimize isolation exercises, since this system favors multi-joint, compound exercises.

**Exercises to minimize include:**

- **Flys and Lateral Raises**
- **Leg Extensions and Leg Curls**

Finally, the Hardgainer Method does not advocate exercising the posterior (rear) deltoid, since pressing movements for the shoulders and chest, and rowing exercises for the back, will increase shoulder development sufficiently.

Here's an example of a typical Hardgainer full-body workout:

## Hardgainer Full-Body Workout

| | |
|---|---|
| Crunches | 1 x failure |
| Squat | 2 x 20 reps |
| Stiff-Leg Deadlift | 1 x 10 |
| Bench Press | 2 x 6 |
| Bent-over Barbell Row | 2 x 8 |
| Military Press | 1 x 6 |
| Barbell Curl | 1 x 6 |
| Standing Calf Raise | 1 x 15 |
| Crunches | 1 x failure |
| Cardio work | 30 minutes |

Perform this workout twice per week, with a 10-20 minute warm-up on a piece of cardio equipment (treadmill, stepper, bike, etc.) at low intensity. Each exercise should also include 1-3 warm-up sets—the workout listed above only specifies the actual full-intensity (to failure) working sets.

Here's an example of a typical Hardgainer split-workout routine:

## Hardgainer Split-Workout

| MONDAY | |
| --- | --- |
| Deadlifts | 3 x 6 reps |
| Incline Bench Press | 3 x 6 |
| Weighted Crunches | 3 x 12 |
| Cardio | 30 minutes |
| **WEDNESDAY** | |
| Lat Pulldowns | 3 x 6 reps |
| Barbell Curls | 2 x 6 |
| Standing Calf Raises | 2 x 15 |
| **Crunches** | 1 x failure |
| FRIDAY | |
| Leg Presses | 1 x 8, 2 x 12 reps |
| Weighted Dips | 2 x 6 |
| Military Press | 3 x 6 |
| Seated Calf Raises | 2 x 20 |
| Cardio | 30 minutes |

Again, the workout would begin with a 10-20 minute warm-up on the treadmill, stepper, or bike at low intensity. Each exercise would also have 1-3 warm-up sets.

# Six Hardgainer Workout Frameworks

In *Beyond Brawn*, McRobert expands on his original full-body and split workouts, presenting six Hardgainer workout frameworks to use as starting points. The frameworks he describes include:

- **Full-Body**
- **Twice Per Week/Divided**
- **Three Times Per Week/Divided**
- **Twice per Week/3-Day Divided**
- **Super Abbreviated/2-Day Divided**
- **Super Abbreviated/Full-Body**

Let's look at the details of each.

## Hardgainer Full-Body Workout (updated)

- General warm-up
- Squat
- Dips
- Stiff-Leg Deadlift
- Dumbbell Press
- Pulldown or pull-up
- Barbell curl
- Calf work
- Crunches

## Hardgainer Twice per Week, Divided Workout

| MONDAY | THURSDAY |
| --- | --- |
| Warm-up | Warm-up |
| Squat | Sumo deadlift or stiff-leg deadlift |
| Bench press or dip | Overhead press |
| Pulldown or row | Curl |
| Calf work | Side Bend |
| Back extension | Neck work |
| Crunches | Side laterals |
| Grip work | Cool down |
| Cool down | |

## Hardgainer Three Times per week, Divided Workout

| MONDAY | WEDNESDAY | FRIDAY |
| --- | --- | --- |
| Warm-up | Warm-up | Warm-up |
| Squat | Calf work | Bench press or dips |
| Stiff-leg deadlift | Crunches | Overhead press |
| Pulldown or row | Grip work | Cool down |
| Cool down | Side Bend | |
| | Curl | |
| | Neck work | |
| | Side laterals | |
| | Cool down | |

# Hardgainer Twice per Week, 3-Day Divided Workout

| Week 1 | Week 2 |
|---|---|
| **MONDAY** | **MONDAY** |
| General warm-up | General warm-up |
| Squat | Leg press |
| Bench press or parallel bar dip | Machine pullover or incline shrug |
| Pulldown or one-arm dumbbell row | Back extension |
| Standing calf work | Barbell curl |
| Crunches | Reverse crunch |
| Grip work | Grip work |
| Cool down | Seated calf work |
|  | Cool down |
| **THURSDAY** | **THURSDAY** |
| General warm-up | Same as Monday of Week 1 |
| Stiff-legged deadlift |  |
| Overhead lockouts |  |
| Dumbbell curl |  |
| Side bend |  |
| Neck work |  |
| Side laterals |  |
| Finger extensions |  |
| Cool down |  |

## Hardgainer Super-Abbreviated Workouts

| Two-Day Divided | |
| --- | --- |
| DAY 1 | DAY 2 |
| General warm-up | General warm-up |
| Bench press or parallel bar dip | Stiff-legged deadlift |
| Overhead press | Pulldown or pull-ups |
| Cool down | Cool down |
| **Full Body** | |
| ROUTINE 1 | ROUTINE 2 |
| General warm-up | General warm-up |
| Squat | Deadlift |
| Parallel bar dip | Bench press or incline press |
| Prone row | Pull-ups |
| Cool down | Cool down |

In the Hardgainer Method, advanced trainers can opt to use specialization training to improve a lagging muscle group, or to improve the performance of a selected exercise. In general, perform the specialization exercises on one training day, and work all other exercises on a separate training day.

Here's an example of how to incorporate Hardgainer specialization training into your workout schedule:

**Monday**
Exercises for the targeted body part or specific exercise to improve

**Thursday**
Exercises for all other body parts.

Finally, note that the Hardgainer and HIT methodologies are very similar, but contain subtle differences. Both use low volume—however; Hardgainer concentrates on cycling the intensity while HIT keeps the intensity high all the time, using a variety of intensity techniques (drop sets, forced reps, etc.).

McRobert used a classification system allowing men to assess their progress using the Hardgainer Method based on total poundage lifted in three core exercises (squat, bench press, and deadlift):

| Classification for Hard-Gaining Men (ages 25-35) Total Weight Lifted (Squat, Bench Press, Deadlift) | | | | |
|---|---|---|---|---|
| | Body Weight | | | |
| | 120 lbs. | 150 lbs. | 180 lbs. | 210 lbs. |
| Very Good | 700 | 850 | 1,025 | 1,200 |
| Terrific | 775 | 950 | 1,150 | 1,325 |
| Outstanding | 875 | 1,075 | 1,300 | 1,500 |

# SuperSlow

In 1982, Ken Hutchins, an employee of Nautilus, was assigned by Arthur Jones to supervise the Nautilus-sponsored Osteoporosis Study at the University of Florida College of Medicine. While there, Hutchins developed the SuperSlow training system as an exercise protocol designed to minimize injury and make exercising safer—while increasing intensity. It's a repetition system designed to make exercise harder and safer—at the same time. SuperSlow is considered a subset or derivative of the High-Intensity Training system, since Arthur Jones concentrated on intensity over form (and allowed loose form when needed), while Hutchins emphasized repetition form as the basis for intensity.

## SuperSlow

- Proper form is essential (no loose form allowed at any time)

- Minimal acceleration, minimal momentum and constant speed during lifting

- Constant tension on the muscle while lifting (Time Under Tension)

- Use 6-12 seconds to lift the weight and the same to lower it

In most weight training systems, you increase the difficulty of the exercise by increasing the weight, typically increasing the acceleration speed in the process. Faster acceleration increases the force applied to the body and can make the exercise more dangerous, especially as you start handling some truly heavy poundages. In other words, Hutchins felt that most training systems make exercises more challenging by making them more dangerous. This holds true with cardiovascular training as well—going from walking to jogging to running to sprinting causes the intensity of the exercise to increase, the forces applied to the body to increase, and the injury potential to increase. It's easier to lose control of your car when you are going 100 mph versus 10 mph. A small shift in the steering wheel at 100 mph often produces disastrous results. Similarly, when you are squatting 400+ pounds, getting out of your groove (your form becomes looser) can potentially cause bad things to happen to your knees, lower back, obliques, etc.

## Force = Mass x <u>Acceleration</u>

Hutchins theorized that if force caused exercise-induced injury, you should strive to minimize force during exercise. Since force is determined by mass times acceleration, and Hutchins discovered that mass could only be reduced slightly before muscular adaptation failed to occur, then acceleration would have to be reduced. (You'll note that his thought process and subsequent derivation of the SuperSlow protocol goes completely against almost all other systems which advocate the use of explosive movements, especially with basic, compound exercises. But remember, his goal was safe training, while others relegate safety to common sense use of form, as appropriate.)

Most individuals have a natural tendency to accelerate when lifting weights, since this makes the exercise easier due to minimized loading on the target muscle(s).

Subsequently, Hutchins realized that minimal acceleration during weightlifting required smooth, constant movement. In his research, he discovered that constant movement could only be accomplished by lifting a weight during a 6-12 second interval—any slower and the movement becomes a series of stops and starts, creating a series of accelerations. At constant speeds, acceleration during lifting is almost eliminated. The goal is to use the slowest speed that produces the smoothest movement possible, in both the eccentric (lifting) and concentric (lowering) portions of the exercise, thereby continuously exposing the target muscle(s) to maximum time-under-tension loads.

Of course, by minimizing acceleration, and keeping constant tension on the working muscle(s), the amount of weight (mass) you are able to lift will be less than normal. Remember, Bill Pearl said you can't lift as much weight as you can throw around.

You can apply SuperSlow to your current workout regimen by simply doing all of your exercises with absolutely strict form, taking 6-12 seconds to lift the weight and the same amount of time to lower it. Of course, since it'll take more time to perform your sets this way, you may want decrease the total number of sets you perform in your workout—otherwise, you may be in the gym for hours (you can work out hard or long, but not both). I would suggest starting out by cutting the number of sets you do for each exercise in half and see how that goes. Remember, applying SuperSlow to your entire workout is entirely different (and produces different overall results) than applying the super-slow technique (Weider's Continuous Tension) to select exercises or sets. That's also valuable and worth a try as well, especially if you just want to sample this technique within your current workout.

# Holistic Training

Dr. Fred Hatfield is first and foremost a powerlifter—a world record powerlifter. In 1980, he set the world record in the squat in the 90kg (198 lbs.) weight class with a lift of 826lbs—a record that still stands today. He wasn't too shabby in other competitive lifts as well, benching over 500lbs and deadlifting over 700lbs in various competitions in the 1980s. As a powerlifter, Hatfield used periodization to improve his lifts. However, his association with Joe Weider and subsequent columnist duties in *Muscle & Fitness* magazine led to his application of periodization principles to bodybuilding. The result was Holistic Training.

Holistic Training centers on the science of muscle cells, where muscles are composed of distinct types of structures. In his book, *Scientific Bodybuilding*, Hatfield (aka "Dr. Squat") describes these components of a muscle cell, their relative sizes, and the best methods to overload each component. All of these components occupy physical space—therefore contributing to the overall size of a muscle. This concept of constructing specific workouts in order to provide overload to each muscle cell component *within a single workout* was the final compression of the periodization cycle from months to weeks to a single session. Behind all the science, Holistic Training is a fancy name for making sure you use the complete array of rep ranges in each workout in order to completely exhaust all the various types of muscles fibers, ensuring that all of them grow to maximum potential.

### Holistic Training

- Use a variety of training methods, rep schemes and speed

- Use a variety of rep ranges (3-5, 6-10, 15+) for power, size and endurance

- Include high-speed, high-rep movements (15+ reps)

- Also perform high-reps with slow, continuous tension

Here are the major muscle cell components, in order from largest to smallest, as a percentage of overall muscle cell size, and the most effective rep ranges and method of performance for overloading them:

## Muscle Cell Components

| Component | % of Cell's Total Size | Method of Overload |
|---|---|---|
| Myofibrils | 20%-30% | 6-12 reps (high-speed) |
| Mitochondria | 15%-25% | 15-25 reps (60% 1RM) at slow speed, continuous tension |
| Sarcoplasm | 20%-30% | 6-25 reps |
| Capillaries | 3%-5% | 15-25 reps at slow speed, continuous tension |
| Fat deposits | 10%-15% | Rest and diet |
| Glycogen | 2%-5% | Diet |
| Connective tissue | 2%-3% | 6-12 reps |
| Sub-cellular substances | 4%-7% | 6-25 reps + rest and diet |

Based on the components of each muscle cell, Holistic Training revolves around two key concepts:

**Each muscle cell component responds to a different form of stress—** therefore each training session should include each method of overload for every muscle group trained.

**Continual adaptation of muscle cell components requires greater amounts of stress** (Selye's Overload and SAID general principles of weight training).

Hatfield's basic Holistic Training workout schema, which he called **ABC training**, consisted of:

- Sets of 4-6 reps done explosively      (muscular power)
- Sets of 12-15 reps done rhythmically    (muscular size)
- Sets of 30+ reps done slowly         (muscular endurance)

The 30 rep sets should take you at least one minute to complete—if it's any shorter, you're lifting too fast. Shoot for one to two minutes per set. Within this schema, you can see the combined concepts of HIT, Periodization and SuperSlow.

This type of training was also advocated and practiced by 8-time Mr. Olympia Lee Haney, particularly during his early 1990s television show on ESPN ("Lee Haney's Championship Workout") where he constantly preached about performing certain exercises explosively and others rhythmically, with differing rep ranges. Typically, basic compound movements such as squats, rows, deadlifts and presses are done explosively for lower reps, while isolation exercises (curls, pushdowns, laterals, extensions) are done rhythmically for higher reps. (Haney and Hatfield went on to conduct numerous joint-seminars on Holistic Training, eventually successfully applying it to the training of world heavyweight champion boxer, Evander Holyfield.)

To get you started, here are some examples of Holistic Training workouts that I've done over the past two decades. Typically, I like to pick a basic, compound movement done with a barbell for the first exercise, followed by a dumbbell or cable movement for the rhythmic portion (cables are especially good for this), ending with an exercise that won't fatigue the lower back—unless I'm targeting the lower back. You don't have to follow this exact schema—try mixing things up every so often, placing the explosive movement in the middle or end. Muscular endurance movements with high reps are also good to warm the muscle(s) up for subsequent exercises.

## Back

- Bent-over Barbell Rows      5-8 reps, explosive
- Pull-downs, any variation      10-15 reps, rhythmically
- Seated Cable Rows      20+ reps, slowly

## Biceps

- Barbell Curls      5-8 reps, explosive
- Dumbbell Curls      10-15 reps, rhythmically
- Cable Curls      20+ reps, slowly

You have to be careful with calves—start with medium and high-rep exercises first. You don't want to initiate explosive movements with cold calves (that Achilles tendon takes about a year to fully heal if ruptured). Get them warmed up first with the other types of movements.

## Calves

- Standing Calf Raises      10-15 reps, rhythmically
- Donkey Calf Raises      5-8 reps, explosive
- Seated Calf Raises      20+ reps, slowly

## Chest

- Barbell Bench Press (any angle) 5-8 reps, explosive
- Dumbbell Flys, any angle      10-15 reps, rhythmically
- Cable Crossovers      20+ reps, slowly

Like calves, be careful with hamstrings—start with a medium or high-rep exercise first to stretch and warm them up. Pull a hamstring (or worse) and you'll be susceptible to that injury for the rest of your life.

## Hamstrings

- Leg Curls, any type      10-15 reps, rhythmically
- Stiff-Leg/Romanian Deadlift      5-8 reps, explosive
- Dumbbell Leg Curls      20+ reps, slowly

## Quads

- Squats, any type      5-8 reps, explosive
- Leg Press      10-15 reps, rhythmically
- Leg Extensions      20+ reps, slowly

For shoulders, you have three options for laterals (front, side, rear). Pick one of those for the slow, cable-based endurance movement. Each time you work your shoulders, rotate another lateral movement into that endurance position.

## Shoulders

- Military Press      5-8 reps, explosive
- Dumbbell Laterals, any type      10-15 reps, rhythmically
- Cable Laterals, any type      20+ reps, slowly

## Traps

- Barbell Shrugs      5-8 reps, explosive
- Upright Rows      10-15 reps, rhythmically
- Cable/Smith Machine Shrugs      20+ reps, slowly

## Triceps

- Close-Grip Bench Press      5-8 reps, explosive
- Extensions      10-15 reps, rhythmically
- Pushdowns      20+ reps, slowly

# Power Factor Training

Peter Sisco developed Power Factor Training in the late 1980s as an attempt to quantify muscular intensity and overload by measuring two indices, the **power factor** and **power index**, to determine the selection of exercises, weights, sets, reps and rep speed that will produce maximal results. Think of this type of training as partials with a purpose.

> ### Power Factor Training
>
> - Compound exercises
> - Maximal weights
> - Partial reps
> - Limited range of motion

The **Power Factor (PF)** is a measurement of the intensity of muscular overload during an exercise, defined as:

$$\text{Power Factor} = (\text{Weight} \times \text{Reps}) \div \text{Time}$$

Here's an example. Let's say you perform 10 reps of bench presses with 200 pounds in one minute. According to the formula above, your Power Factor on that exercises is 2,000 pounds per minute. Now, during a future workout you manage to perform those 10 reps with the same weight in only 30 seconds. Your Power Factor is now 4,000 pounds per minute. You just increased the intensity—by a measured amount. One of Sisco's goals was to move the weight training world from a subjective state ("yeah, I think that was a lot tougher than last time") to an objective one ("my Power Factor on bench press doubled in the last XX days"). But that's not the whole story here…

You can reach extremely high Power Factor numbers simply by performing certain exercises with very heavy weights for short periods of time. Such as leg presses. If you perform 500 pounds for 5 reps on the leg press in 10 seconds, then your Power Factor would be 15,000 pounds per minute. But realistically, can you keep up that performance for extended periods of time (30 seconds or more)? That's where the Power Index comes in.

The **Power Index (PI)** is a measurement of the duration of a given power factor (how long you can sustain the intensity), defined as:

$$\text{Power Index} = (\text{Weight x Reps}) \times \text{Power Factor} \times 10^{-6}$$

For those mathematically challenged, you can also use the equivalent formula:

$$\text{Power Index} = (\text{Weight x Reps}) \times \text{Power Factor} \div 1{,}000{,}000$$

Using the example above, if you perform 500 pounds for 5 reps on the leg press in 10 seconds, your Power Index would be 37.5. This number reflects both your intensity and the duration you were able to sustain that intensity.

Lifters record their power indices for each workout and attempt to increase it on subsequent workouts. In order to increase your power factor, you must lift more total weight in the same period of time (duration), or the same amount of weight in a shorter period (nothing is performed slow here, let alone SuperSlow). To increase your power index, you must sustain your power factor for a longer period. Performing additional sets can accomplish this. Typically, the number of sets performed varies with the weight trainer's level of experience. For example, beginners typically perform one set of each exercise, while intermediate trainees perform 1-3 sets and advanced trainers perform 3-5 sets.

Sisco noted that certain types of training and specific types of exercises produced higher power factors and indices for most lifters. These styles of training and core exercises form the basis of Power Factor Training. Let's take a more in-depth look.

# Power Factor Training Style

## Partial Reps (Target Range of Motion)

Partial reps are recommended because more reps can be performed in a given period of time versus full-range reps. The partial reps should approximate the last two to four inches of the range of motion for the muscle(s) under stress. For example, when you perform partial reps in the bench press, only lower and press the weight two to four inches from the lockout position. Overhead presses and leg presses are handled in the same manner.

## Limited Range of Motion

The partial reps are performed in their strongest range of motion, allowing you to use as much weight as possible. For example, in the squat you are strongest near the fully upright position, therefore with partial reps you can use weights in excess of your 1RM and only lower the weight a quarter of the way down (quarter squats) and then push it back up.

## Compound Exercises

Exercises that involve multi-joint movements are preferred over isolation exercises since more weight can be handled. For example, since you can use heavy weights, a common compound movement for working the chest is the traditional bench press. Exercises that don't allow such heavy weights (dumbbell flys) are left as isolation exercises. Not surprisingly, when using maximal weights with these compound exercises, the power rack is your friend.

A typical Power Factor training program would include two alternating workouts ("Workout A" and "Workout B"), where each workout includes five to six exercises. The number of sets per exercise varies, depending on your skill level and recovery ability. Beginners to this type of training should perform one set of each exercise, while intermediates can perform 1-3 sets, and advanced trainers can perform 3-5 sets.

Here's a typical Power Factor alternating workout program categorized by muscle group:

| Workout A | Workout B |
|-----------|-----------|
| Shoulders | Lower Back |
| Traps | Chest |
| Triceps | Upper Back |
| Biceps | Quads |
| Abs | Hamstrings |
| | Calves |

You'll notice these workouts alternate the pushing and pulling muscle groups of the body, which also helps you use max weights.

Here are some example Power Factor workouts to get you started. For exercises performed in the power rack, set the safety rails so that you can really pile on the weight, even if that limits the range of motion you are accustomed to.

## Workout A

- Standing Barbell Military Press (in power rack)
- Barbell Shrugs
- Close-Grip Bench Press (in power rack)
- Barbell Curls
- Weighted sit-ups or crunches

## Workout B

- Deadlifts
- Bench Press (in power rack)
- Bent-over Barbell Row
- Squats (in power rack)
- Stiff-Leg or Romanian Deadlifts
- Standing Calf Raises

The next time you're in the gym and notice a guy doing quarter squats or half presses, he might just be following the Power Factor Training methodology. Sure. At least when you do it and someone asks, "hey, why don't you lower the bar all the way down?" you'll have an intelligent answer for them.

# Positions of Flexion (POF)

Steve Holman, former editor of *Ironman* magazine, developed the Positions of Flexion weight training system in the early 1990s, based on the concept of multi-angular training, where each muscle is maximally stressed from three different angular positions within the same workout. (It also helped sell more *Ironman* magazines.)

## Positions of Flexion

Work each muscle from the 3 angular positions within the same workout

The three angular positions, the positions of flexion, include:

- **The Midrange**
- **The Stretch**
- **The Contraction**

Let's look at each of the positions in detail.

## The Midrange

Midrange movements, where the muscle is neither fully stretched or contracted, activate the majority of the muscle fibers, using basic exercises such as squats, bench presses, curls, etc. These are the heart and soul of most traditional weight lifting workouts.

## The Stretch

Maximizes the stress on the target muscle at the point where it is completely stretched, such as flys for the pectorals, or incline curls or preacher curls for the biceps.

## The Contraction

Maximizes the stress on the target muscle at a point where the muscle is fully contracted, such as leg extensions for the quadriceps or concentration curls for the biceps.

Here's a brief list of exercises by muscle group for each of the three angular positions:

## Abs

- *Midrange:*       Knee-ups
- *Stretch:*        Cable Crunches
- *Contraction:*    Crunches

## Back

- *Midrange:*       Chins, Pulldowns
- *Stretch:*        Pullovers
- *Contraction:*    Rows

## Biceps

- *Midrange:*       Barbell Curls, Dumbbell Curls
- *Stretch:*        Incline Curls, Preacher Curls
- *Contraction:*    Concentration Curls

## Chest

- *Midrange:*       Bench Press
- *Stretch:*        Flys
- *Contraction:*    Cable Crossovers

## Delts

- *Midrange:*       Dumbbell Presses, Military Presses
- *Stretch:*        Behind the Back Cable Laterals
- *Contraction:*    Seated Dumbbell Laterals, Bent-over Dumbbell Laterals

## Hamstrings

- *Midrange:*    Stiff-Leg Deadlifts
- *Stretch:*    Stiff-Leg Deadlifts, Leg Curls
- *Contraction:*    Leg Curls

## Quadriceps

- *Midrange:*    Squats, Leg Presses
- *Stretch:*    Sissy Squats
- *Contraction:*    Leg Extensions

## Triceps

- *Midrange:*    Close-Grip Bench Press
- *Stretch:*    Overhead Extensions
- *Contraction:*    Kickbacks

Larry Scott, two-time Mr. Olympia, famous for his legendary biceps, used the positions of flexion concept in the 1960s before it had a name. His popularized bicep workout (discussed in *Loaded Guns*) exemplified this approach, consisting of midrange dumbbell curls on the preacher bench, followed by strict full-range barbell preacher curls, finishing with reverse E-Z bar preacher curls. The workout often included Spider Curls for the contraction movement.

The ever-popular barbell 21's exercise, where you perform 21 total reps, seven reps each in the bottom half, top half and full range of the curl are another prime example of angular training. This concept can be applied to many other exercises as well, including leg curls and extensions, laterals, and presses.

It's pretty easy to incorporate Positions of Flexion training into your workout—just select one exercise from each of the three positions for the muscle group you are training. Most of the time you'll start with the midrange movement, since it's typically a basic mass-building exercise, followed by either the stretch or contraction movements—however, experiment with different sequences (stretch/ contraction/midrange , contraction/midrange/stretch) and don't be afraid to mix things up to keep your body adapting.

# Static Contraction Training

What's old is new again. What was popularized in the 1930s with Charles Atlas and the "Dynamic-Tension" workout—so you wouldn't get sand kicked in your face—came full circle in the 1990s with Peter Sisco's publication of *Static Contraction Training*. This led to the current Functional Isometric movement in training today. For all those years in between, isometric-based contraction training never went away—it was just renamed, from "isometrics" to "isotonics" (later combined as "isometronics"), to "functional isometric contractions". Even the Europeans jumped in with "auxotonics".

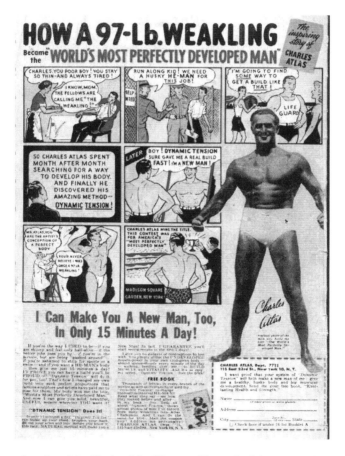

*A version of the Charles Atlas "Dynamic Tension" ad that appeared in magazines and comic books for over 50 years*

Static Contraction Training emphasizes workout intensity through the use of extremely heavy weights and a very limited range of motion, rather than focusing on the frequency and volume of exercise.

## Static Contraction Training

- **Heavy weights**
- **Very limited or no range of motion**
- **Effort based on Time Under Load—not reps**

This type of training does not use the traditional system of repetitions—instead, it only deals with isometric contraction for 5-10 seconds, using the heaviest weight you can handle in the strongest range of motion for a particular movement. This is the range where individuals can handle the most weight and are least susceptible to injury. It may take one or two workouts to determine the correct weights and range of motion for each exercise under this system. However, once you discover this, you simply employ the principle of progressive overload—either increase the weight used for the contractions, the time each contraction is held, or both. Remember: no repetitions—only record the time under load (TUL).

Also, note that Static Contraction Training often requires the assistance of a spotter in order to help you move the weight into position. If you don't have a spotter, the power rack or Smith Machine becomes very useful for this type of training.

So, how does Static Contraction Training work in practice? Let's look at a common scenario.

If you normally bench press 225lbs. for 6-8 reps, you might select 275lbs. for your static contraction weight, holding the loaded bar approximately 2-3 inches below the lockout position for 5-10 seconds. As you accustom to this type of training, you may be amazed at some of the poundages you are able to use in near lockout position. John Grimek, perhaps the greatest bodybuilder from the 1930s and 1940s, famously described performing static presses with a 1000lb barbell hanging from the beams in his parent's basement. During one training session, the barbell slipped from the chain it was hanging from and almost brought the house down. You don't have to take things to that extreme.

Powerlifters have used isometric-type training like this for years—they often call it "pin pressing", where they press the bar against the top pins in a power rack with as much force as possible for 6-8 seconds. Additionally, many martial arts practitioners, including Bruce Lee, as well as Indian yogis have used this form of training for centuries to increase size and strength. Bruce Lee was known to hold a 135lb. barbell out in front of his face with straight arms for several seconds.

Notice that Static Contraction Training and Power Factor Training are closely related by the limited range of motion each uses. The primary difference is that Power Factor Training moves the weight through a strong-range partial (e.g., limited range of motion) for a number of reps, while Static Contraction Training does not move the weight at all, does not use reps, and only employs muscle contraction within a strong range position.

Not surprisingly, since these two training systems are similar, they also share a common workout regimen of recommending five to six exercises per workout, organized into two alternating sessions ("Workout A", "Workout B") as listed below:

| Workout A | Workout B |
| --- | --- |
| Shoulders | Lower Back |
| Traps | Chest |
| Triceps | Upper Back |
| Biceps | Quads |
| Abs | Hamstrings |
| | Calves |

Based on these regimens, here are some Static Contraction workouts to get you started. Since you will be using very heavy weights with little to no range of motion, I recommend you perform all of these exercises in the power rack or Smith Machine, setting the safety rails/latches appropriately so that you don't kill yourself.

## Workout A

- Standing Barbell Military Press
- Barbell Shrugs
- Close-Grip Bench Press
- Barbell Curls (bottom or top of movement—set the safeties appropriately)
- Weighted sit-ups or crunches

## Workout B

- Good Mornings (set the safeties so you only lift the bar an inch or two)
- Bench Press (set the safeties so you work specific areas—start, mid-point, lockout)
- Weighted Chins (hold yourself at various places in the range of motion—top, mid-point)
- Leg Curls (work the start, mid-point, and contracted positions)
- Standing Calf Raises (get as high up on your toes as possible and hold)

Again, the number of sets to perform per exercise varies, depending on your skill level and recovery ability. It's advised that beginners to this type of training perform one set of each exercise, intermediates perform 1-3 sets, and advanced trainers can perform 3-5 sets.

Finally, the Static Contraction Training system recommends that the frequency of workouts be no more than two times per week for the first 6-8 workouts, then be reduced to once per week, in order to avoid over-training.

Critics of Static Contraction Training have emphasized that it only develops strength at the point being worked. However, further research has shown that isometrics produce strength gains at 15 degrees plus or minus the angle worked. This is valuable information for those who wish to increase their strength and muscular development with squats, presses and rows, especially if (when) you hit a plateau. It's also why Power Factor Training and Positions of Flexion produce results.

Larry Scott, the first Mr. Olympia in 1966, also used static contraction isometrics when building his shoulder width. Born with a relatively narrow shoulder structure, Larry was determined to find a method that would allow him to pack as much muscle as possible on his side deltoids. Here's one of the things he did. Immediately after completing a set of side dumbbell laterals, Larry would pick up a set of dumbbells roughly twice the weight he just used, lifting and holding them out to the side as long as possible. You can also use this technique at the end of other exercises, such as leg extensions and curls, seated barbell curls, and many others.

Here are more exercises that are especially well-suited for static contractions:

## Abs

- **Leg Raises** – hold your legs just below the mid-point for as long as possible

## Back

- **Seated Cable Rows, Machine Rows, Chins, Pulldowns** – hold the weight in the fully contracted position

## Biceps

- **Any type of curl** – hold at the mid-point (where your forearm is parallel to the floor)

## Calves

- **Any type of calf raise or press** – hold the weight in the fully contracted position

## Chest

- **Presses** – use the "pin pressing" technique described earlier or hold the bar in the lockout or near-lockout position
- **Flys** – hold the fly position at mid-point (this works well if you only have access to dumbbells)

## Hamstrings

- **Leg Curls** – hold the weight in the fully contracted position as well as the mid-point

## Quadriceps

- **Squats** – hold the weight just below the lockout position (use a power rack or Smith Machine for this)

## Shoulders

- **Presses** – use the same technique as chest presses
- **Laterals** – hold the weight at the mid-point or as close to the mid-point as possible

## Trapezius

- **Shrugs** – hold the weight in the fully contracted position as well as the fully extended position

## Triceps

- **Close-Grip Presses** – use the same technique as chest presses
- **Pushdowns** – hold the weight in the fully contracted position as well as at the mid-point

Note that you can perform static contractions at either the beginning or end of your set. If using them at the beginning, perform the static hold for your desired length of time, then immediately perform a regular set of full range movement with your regular training weight.

Finally, Static Contraction Training is useful in an overall program for recovering from an injury, especially those that involve the shoulder. For example, let's assume one of your shoulders is temporarily injured (we're not talking about chronic injuries here), preventing you from performing full range presses. After a period of rest, you can start training your shoulders by performing static holds with presses in a power rack or Smith Machine.

Eventually, you should be able to work to partial presses, and then full range presses. Of course, in these cases you should start with lighter weights, slowly working your way up to max poundages as your injury heals.

# Final Thoughts

By now, you should have a good understanding of various ideologies and methods for lifting weights to maximize your muscular growth. It's eye-opening to witness the vast array of philosophies, techniques and methods that can be applied to barbells and dumbbells.

Well known strength coach Dan John has repeatedly said that "anything works for 3-4 weeks, but nothing works forever". If you try any of the weight training systems in this book for the first time, they are bound to work. The real key is to find which one or combination of them works best for you. Your body presents an inner universe that only you can discover and master. That takes hard work, consistency and time, but the knowledge you gain will last a lifetime. Your goal is to keep adapting and the overall lesson here is that change is good.

# References

Please consult the following books if you want to read more about each of the weight training systems presented here.

**Brawn** (Stuart McRobert)

**Beyond Brawn: The Insider's Encyclopedia on How to Build Muscle & Might** (Stuart McRobert)

**The New High-Intensity Training: The Best Muscle Building System You've Never Tried** (Ellington Darden)

**High-Intensity Training the Mike Mentzer Way** (Mike Mentzer and John Little)

**Periodization: Theory and Methodology of Training** (Tudor Bompa and G. Gregory Haff)

**Joe Weider's Ultimate Bodybuilding** (Joe Weider and Bill Reynolds)

**Power Factor Training: A Scientific Approach to Building Lean Muscle Mass** (Peter Sisco and John Little)

**Critical Mass: The Positions-of-Flexion Approach to Explosive Muscle Growth** (Steve Holman)

**Train, eat, grow: The positions-of-flexion muscle-training manual** (Steve Holman)

**Static Contraction Training** (Peter Sisco and John Little)

**An Introduction to Static Contraction Training—The World's Fastest Workout** (Peter Sisco)

# Other Books by this Author

## Supermen: Building Maximum Muscle for a Lifetime

"As an avid weightlifter and a physician specializing in physical medicine and rehabilitation, I found this book to be a well-written, die-hard approach to muscle and fitness. Craig has the uncanny ability to combine the key ingredients of basic muscle physiology, proper techniques, and hard core lifts into a practical, organized and entertaining guide to building muscle. This book is a must read for anyone who is serious about building maximum muscle for a lifetime."

— Dr. Mark Gloth

Made in the USA
San Bernardino, CA
03 June 2014